ATLAS OF
NORMAL FETAL ULTRASONOGRAPHIC ANATOMY

# Atlas of
# Normal Fetal Ultrasonographic Anatomy

## Richard A. Bowerman, M.D.

*Department of Radiology*
*University of Michigan School of Medicine*
*Ann Arbor, Michigan*

YEAR BOOK MEDICAL PUBLISHERS, INC.

CHICAGO

Copyright © 1986 by Year Book Medical Publishers, Inc. All rights reserved. No part of this publication may be reproduced, stored in a retrieval system, or transmitted, in any form or by any means, electronic, mechanical, photocopying, recording, or otherwise, without prior written permission from the publisher. Printed in the United States of America.

0   9   8   7   6   5   4   3   2   1

**Library of Congress Cataloging in Publication Data**

Bowerman, Richard A.
  Atlas of normal fetal ultrasonographic anatomy.
  Bibliography: p.
  Includes index.
  1. Ultrasonics in obstetrics—Atlases.  2. Fetus—
Physiology—Atlases.  3. Fetus—Abnormalities—Diagnosis.
4. Diagnosis, Ultrasonic.  I. Title.  [DNLM:  1. Fetus—
anatomy & histology—atlases.  2. Ultrasonic Diagnosis—
atlases.  WQ 17 B786a]
RG527.5.U48B68   1986        618.3′207′543        85-14222
ISBN 0-8151-1104-5

Sponsoring Editor: James D. Ryan, Jr.
Manager, Copyediting Services: Frances M. Perveiler
Production Project Manager: R. Allen Reedtz
Proofroom Supervisor: Shirley E. Taylor

# Preface

IMPROVED INSTRUMENTATION has extended the role of ultrasound in obstetrics beyond the determination of gestational age, placental and fetal position, detection of multiple gestations, complications of pregnancy, and gross congenital malformations. Technical advances in ultrasonic instrumentation, particularly the advent of high resolution real-time scanners, have provided a means for detailed identification of normal fetal anatomy. Similarly, earlier and more subtle diagnoses of fetal structural abnormalities are now routinely made. The inherent flexibility of real-time sonography is essential to sonographic evaluation of the normal and abnormal fetus. The diagnostic accuracy of fetal sonography is highly operator dependent. Even a skilled and experienced ultrasonographer, dedicated to a thorough evaluation of the fetus, requires significant scanning time to confirm normalcy or detect variances from normal.

Increased diagnostic capability to identify multiple structural lesions within the fetus has many implications. Early diagnosis of a congenital anomaly with a hopeless prognosis allows for termination of pregnancy. Detection of a less severe defect or late determination of severe malformation may alter the subsequent obstetrical course. Certain mass lesions may preclude vaginal delivery in order to preserve fetal and/or maternal integrity. Caesarean section may also be indicated when continued intrauterine existence is detrimental to fetal well-being. Some malformations may be followed to a normal term delivery, with subsequent extrauterine evaluation and therapy. It is imperative that a fetus with a significant anomaly be delivered at a medical facility where the appropriate surgical and medical specialists are available for prompt treatment of the neonate so as to avoid further postnatal complications.

Identification of the malformed fetus is predicated on a strong knowledge of the sonographic appearance of normal fetal anatomy. Both false positive and false negative diagnoses of fetal malformation may have far-reaching medical, psychological, and even medicolegal implications. To this end, normal sonographic fetal anatomy is extensively presented in a combined body region/systems approach, as one would systematically image the fetus. A brief section is included on the functional evaluation of the developing fetus. Recognition of certain pitfalls in the evaluation of fetal anatomy is addressed in appropriate sections.

An extensive bibliography has been included for those individuals who desire information beyond that which is feasible in an atlas format.

This volume is intended as a comprehensive and unified source of reference detailing normal sonographic fetal anatomy for the ever-increasing multiplicity of medical personnel involved with fetal sonography.

RICHARD A. BOWERMAN, M.D.

# Contents

# CHAPTER 1

# Fetal Scanning

## INDICATIONS

During the course of an obstetrical ultrasound ordered for any reason, the fetus should be examined for documentation of viability, gestational age, and exclusion of major anatomic defects of the head, spine, trunk, and extremities.

Certain populations have specific indications for directed sonographic examination of the fetus, based on a higher than average probability of fetal abnormality. These indications fall into the following areas:

a. An elevation in the maternal serum or amniotic fluid alpha-fetoprotein. This is most frequently associated with open neural tube defects but may be seen in other instances including fetal demise, multiple gestations, Rh disease, fetal gastrointestinal or renal abnormalities, and Turner's syndrome.

b. A family history of a chromosomal abnormality or other potentially heritable disease which may manifest morphologic changes that could be identified sonographically.

c. An abnormal amniotic fluid volume (patient large or small for dates). Polyhydramnios is associated in particular with neural tube defects (deficient swallowing mechanism) and high gastrointestinal tract obstructions, as well as many other miscellaneous abnormalities. Oligohydramnios results from either a failure of fetal urine production (bilateral nonfunctioning kidneys) or obstruction of excretion (bilateral ureteral or bladder outlet obstruction).

## TECHNIQUE

Sonographic evaluation of the fetus is only one component of the obstetrical ultrasound examination, which also involves evaluation of the placenta, uterus, adnexa, and an estimation of fluid volume. The order of examination is not critical as long as a complete study is accomplished. However, the potential for fetal movement and positional changes suggests that fetal imaging be performed whenever visualization of the desired structures is optimal.

### Patient Preparation

The gravid uterus tends to displace bowel out of the pelvis and lower abdomen, creating its own window for visualizing uterine contents. The maternal bladder should be distended for adequate visualization of the cervix and lower uterine segment as a general part of the obstetrical examination and will frequently be necessary to image low-lying fetal parts.

### Equipment

While static or articulated arm "contact" scanning provides a global view of uterine size, placental location, fluid volume, and fetal position, real-time scanning is required for an adequate fetal examination. Persistent and rapid fetal movement is frequent, particularly through the first 20 weeks, thus dictating the use of real-time instrumentation with its inherent flexibility. Fetal movements can be observed and appropriate adjustment in transducer orientation rapidly accomplished to image the desired anatomy. The quality of real-time instrumentation varies dramatically; however, constant technological advances insure an ever increasing ability to image the fetus in utero. Either sector scan or linear array transducers may be used, each with its own advantages and disadvantages. Sector scanners may prove more useful for deeply positioned fetuses, where a wide field of view is necessary distally and a narrow field of view proximally is no detriment. Linear array scanners provide the advantage of a wider overall field of view, this being of particular value for the more superficially positioned fetus. Occasionally, a small head sector scan transducer is necessary for scanning access in confined areas, such as with a low-lying fetus.

## Fetal Orientation and Position Determination

Initial scanning of the uterine contents should be performed transversely and longitudinally to determine the lie of the fetus, which is generally cephalic, breech, or occasionally transverse in the first half of pregnancy. Once the longitudinal axis of the fetus within the uterus is defined, a 90-degree rotation to the fetal transverse plane will delineate the orientation of the spine, and define the right and left sides of the fetus. The approximate position of the extremities will be suggested by knowing the fetal lie and spinal orientation. Subsequent transverse scanning to the level of the pelvis or upper thorax will delineate the adjacent extremities which then can be individually scanned by following the known bony landmarks distally. As considerable fetal motion may occur during the course of an examination, reassessment of fetal lie and position may be intermittently necessary to confirm appropriate imaging planes.

## Limitations

As with any ultrasound examination, maternal obesity will adversely affect image quality. Incomplete maternal bladder filling and certain fetal positions may hinder complete fetal examination, particularly when portions of the bony skeleton obscure underlying soft tissues. Fetal motion, when extreme, lengthens examination time by necessitating constant transducer adjustment and may preclude identification and documentation of certain structures. In such instances, a videotape examination may prove useful. With oligohydramnios, fetal structures are compressed together and against the uterus and may be held in unusual positions. Both of these factors make fetal examination difficult in part because the natural contrast between adjacent structures provided by intervening amniotic fluid is not present.

## Practical Scanning Hints

If the fetus is in a position which precludes adequate evaluation, several maneuvers may be tried. Maternal positional changes, i.e., Trendelenburg, decubitus, walking, etc., may stimulate fetal motion. Occasionally, partial or complete emptying of the bladder may lead to improved fetal position; however, this should not be attempted until the remaining examination, i.e., placenta localization, as much fetal evaluation as possible, etc., is completed, as subsequent visualization may actually be degraded by bladder emptying. Finally, repeat scanning at a later date may reveal improved fetal position.

A relatively systematic examination of the fetus is recommended, and a check list may prove valuable to ensure that no areas are missed. As certain measurements require precise scanning planes (biparietal diameter, abdominal circumference, femur length, etc.), initial scanning might best be directed toward obtaining this data if the fetal position is initially satisfactory. In general, for complete fetal scanning, a regional anatomic approach is suggested. The head is initially scanned for determination of the biparietal diameter and evaluation of general intracranial anatomy, such as an assessment of ventricular size. The appearance of the fetal spine is documented in the longitudinal plane, which also provides orientation for subsequent transverse scanning of the complete spine from the occiput to the coccyx. Especially in the flexible older fetus, transducer orientation on the maternal abdomen will need to be adjusted periodically to maintain a symmetrical transverse section through the fetal spine. Attention should be paid only to the spine as the trunk is scanned transversely, so as not to inadvertently miss viewing a segment while looking elsewhere. Subsequently, transverse imaging through the thorax and abdomen will assess the other soft tissue and bony structures within the normal confines of the fetal trunk, including cardiac activity (rate and rhythm) and the normal presence of the stomach, umbilical vein, bladder, and possibly gallbladder. A third, separate transverse ''pass'' through the entire head, neck, and trunk should be obtained, specifically looking for masses protruding externally to the cutaneous margins of the fetus.

Finally, the extremities are studied. Individual extremities are identified by their relationship to structures within the trunk, such as the shoulder girdle or ribs for the upper extremities and the iliac crests, ischial spines, or bladder for the lower extremities. Once the appropriate bones are localized, rotation of the transducer will yield longitudinal images for measurement and further orient one for localization of the more distal structures of any individual extremity.

## REFERENCES

Bartrum R.J. Jr., Crow H.C.: Pregnancy, in Bartrum R.J. (ed.): *Real-Time Ultrasound*. Philadelphia, W.B. Saunders Co., 1983, pp. 140–155.

Bowie J.D., Andreotti R.F.: Estimating gestational age in utero, in Callen P.W. (ed.): *Ultrasonography in Obstetrics and Gynecology*. Philadelphia, W.B. Saunders Co., 1983, pp. 21–39.

Garrett W.J.: Fetal organ imaging, in Sabbagha R.E. (ed.): *Diagnostic Ultrasound Applied to Obstetrics and Gynecology*. New York, Harper & Row, 1980, pp. 35–50.

Johnson M.L., Hattan R.A., Rees G.K.: The normal fetus. *Semin. Roentgenol.* 17:182–189, 1982.

Johnson M.L., Rees G.K., Hattan R.A.: Normal fetal anatomy, in Callen P.W. (ed.): *Ultrasonography in Obstetrics and Gynecology*. Philadelphia, W.B. Saunders Co., 1983, pp. 41–59.

Sanders R.C., Miner N.S., Martin J.: Fetal anatomy, in Sanders R.C., James A.E. Jr. (eds.): *The Principles and Practice of Ultrasonography in Obstetrics and Gynecology*. New York, Appleton-Century-Crofts, 1985, pp. 123–159.

# CHAPTER 2

# Fetal Well-Being

## GROWTH AND DEVELOPMENT/FETAL MEASUREMENTS

A major application for obstetrical sonography is in the evaluation of normal fetal growth and development and the exclusion of intrauterine growth retardation. Growth-retarded infants have a poorer long-term prognosis for somatic growth and functional development than do normal-sized neonates. Extensive efforts by multiple investigators attempt to define sonographic criteria for the diagnosis of intrauterine growth retardation. Measurement of the total intrauterine volume, estimation of amniotic fluid volume, and evaluation of the placenta have all been suggested as having complementary roles in this diagnosis.

Multiple fetal measurements both individually and in various combinations and ratios have been suggested as useful in identification of a growth-retarded fetus. These include the biparietal diameter, occipitofrontal diameter, head circumference, transverse abdominal diameter, AP abdominal diameter, abdominal circumference, abdominal area, femur length, fetal weight derived from biparietal diameter and abdominal circumference, head-to-abdomen circumference ratio, femur length-to-abdominal circumference ratio, femur length-to-biparietal diameter ratio, etc. Examples within appropriate chapters illustrate the anatomic landmarks and technique for deriving the indicated individual fetal measurements, and references in this and other chapters explain the detailed application and rationale of the various multifactorial determinations.

## FUNCTIONAL EVALUATION OF THE FETUS

Prior to the advent of real-time ultrasound, maternal observation was the primary means for documenting degree of fetal activity, in an attempt to correlate fetal movement with perinatal outcome. The fetus can now be directly observed with real-time ultrasound not only to evaluate generalized fetal movement, but to discern specific extremity, trunk, head, and neck movements; to document the presence of fetal breathing and swallowing; and to confirm normal cardiac rate and rhythm. In the assessment of fetal well-being, various biophysical profiles have been proposed, including combined documentation of fetal breathing and various extremity movements. While the presence of normal fetal movement and breathing patterns generally suggests a favorable postnatal outcome, the absence of such fetal activity may or may not portend poorly for the fetus, as the various described fetal activities are not constant in nature but rather demonstrate considerable range in frequency.

### Fetal Breathing

Respiratory activity can be observed as early as the late first trimester with simultaneous inward depression of the thorax and outward protrusion of the abdomen. Early respiratory activity is irregular in rate, frequency, and amplitude; however, as pregnancy progresses, a more uniform pattern of fetal breathing emerges with a normal frequency of 12 to 60 times per minute. In the third trimester, an examination over 30 minutes will demonstrate breathing in most all fetuses. Fetal breathing may be affected by certain maternal factors including medications and glucose administration, the latter of which increases breathing activity. Fetal hiccups occur in approximately 2% of fetuses in the third trimester. A hiccup is indicated by a more rapid thrusting of the chest and abdomen in a to-and-fro fashion.

## Fetal Movement

The earliest documented activity within the embryo is that of cardiac motion or flickering seen at approximately 5.5 to 6 weeks gestational age. By 7 to 8 weeks, the embryo can be seen to occasionally move in a somewhat rigid and focal fashion, with embryo/fetal movement progressively increasing until the mid second trimester. By approximately 10 weeks, distinctive fetal movement patterns can be observed with (1) slow, gliding or rolling motions of part or all of the fetus, or (2) a rapid jumping or jerky type motion appearing reflexive in nature. Both of these motions occur spontaneously several times per minute, while the latter, more reflexive type motion may be stimulated by mechanical pressure on the uterus. These early documentations of fetal activity are important in confirming the ongoing presence of a normally developing embryo/fetus. Throughout the second trimester, gross fetal movements of extremities, trunk, head, and neck continue in addition to fine motor activities of various isolated body parts. Within the third trimester, gross fetal motion of major body parts may be seen up to 30 times per hour, and in only 1% of cases will a 45-minute interval without significant fetal activity occur. Such diminished motion suggests the possibility of a neuromuscular abnormality or generalized fetal compromise.

## Fetal Cardiac Activity

Fetal cardiac activity has been documented as early as 5.5 to 6 weeks gestational age as a flicker within the embryo centrally. This will be identified prior to any generalized motion of the embryo. Frequent episodes of sinus bradycardia may be noted particularly within the second trimester, and sinus tachycardia may be noted in the third trimester. Only sustained heart rates of less than 100 or greater than 200 or discrepancies between the ventricular and atrial rates should arouse suspicion of cardiac abnormality. M-mode echocardiography or videotaping are useful in documentation of both normal and abnormal rates and rhythms.

## Fetal Swallowing

Fetal swallowing can be seen through a large portion of the second and third trimester as a normal phenomenon occurring intermittently up to several times per minute. Swallowing plays a role in the normal dynamics of amniotic fluid movement and, when reduced, is associated with polyhydramnios. One can see opening and closing of the mouth, movement of the tongue, and occasional movement in the region of the hypopharynx, all presumed to be associated with fetal swallowing.

REFERENCES

## Growth & Development/Fetal Measurements

Birnholz J.C.: Ultrasound characterization of fetal growth. *Ultrasonic Imaging* 2:135–149, 1900.

Campbell S., Thoms A.: Ultrasound measurement of the fetal head to abdomen circumference ratio in the assessment of growth retardation. *Br. J. Obstet. Gynaecol.* 84:165–174, 1977.

Campbell S., Wilkin D.: Ultrasonic measurement of fetal abdomen circumference in the estimation of fetal weight. *Br. J. Obstet. Gynaecol.* 82:689–697, 1975.

Campogrande M., Todros T., Brizzolara M.: Prediction of birth weight by ultrasound measurements of the fetus. *Br. J. Obstet. Gynaecol.* 84:175–178, 1977.

Crane J.P., Kopta M.M.: Prediction of intrauterine growth retardation via ultrasonically measured head/abdominal circumference ratios. *Obstet. Gynecol.* 54:597–601, 1979.

Depp R.: Dynamics of fetal growth, in Sabbagha R.E. (ed.): *Diagnostic Ultrasound Applied to Obstetrics and Gynecology*. New York, Harper & Row, pp. 111–125, 1980.

Deter R.L., Hadlock F.P., Harrist R.B.: Evaluation of normal fetal growth and the detection of intrauterine growth retardation, in Callen P.W. (ed.): *Ultrasonography in Obstetrics and Gynecology*. Philadelphia, W.B. Saunders Co., pp. 113–140, 1983.

Deter R.L., Hadlock F.P., Harrist R.B., et al.: Evaluation of three methods for obtaining fetal weight estimates using dynamic image ultrasound. *J. C. U.* 9:421–425, 1981.

Deter R.L., Harrist R.B., Hadlock F.P., et al.: The use of ultrasound in the detection of intrauterine growth retardation: a review. *J. C. U.* 10:9–16, 1982.

Deter R.L., Harrist R.B., Hadlock F.P., et al.: Fetal head and abdominal circumferences: II. A critical re-evaluation of the relationship to menstrual age. *J. C. U.* 10:365–372, 1982.

Deter R.L., Harrist R.B., Hadlock F.P., et al.: The use of ultrasound in the assessment of normal fetal growth: a review. *J. C. U.* 9:481–493, 1981.

Gross B.H., Callen P.W., Filly R.A.: The relationship of fetal transverse body diameter and biparietal diameter in the diagnosis of intrauterine growth retardation. *J. Ultrasound Med.* 1:361–365, 1982.

Hadlock F.P., Deter R.L., Harrist R.B., et al.: Computer assisted analysis of fetal age in the third trimester using multiple fetal growth parameters. *J. C. U.* 11:313–316, 1983.

Hadlock F.P., Deter R.L., Harrist R.B., et al.: Estimating fetal age: computer-assisted analysis of multiple fetal growth parameters. *Radiology* 152:497–501, 1984.

Hern W.M.: Correlation of fetal age and measurements between 10 and 26 weeks of gestation. *Obstet. Gynecol.* 63:26–32, 1984.

Jordaan H.V.F.: Estimation of fetal weight by ultrasound. *J. C. U.* 11:59–66, 1983.

Kurtz A.B., Wapner R.J., Kurtz R.J., et al.: Analysis of biparietal diameter as an accurate indicator of gestational age. *J. C. U.* 8:319–326, 1980.

Lunt R., Chard T.: A new method for estimation of fetal weight in late pregnancy by ultrasonic scanning. *Br. J. Obstet. Gynaecol.* 83:1–5, 1976.

O'Brien G.D., Queenan J.T.: Ultrasound fetal femur length in relation to intrauterine growth retardation. *Am. J. Obstet. Gynecol.* 144(pt. 2):35–39, 1982.

Ott W.J., Doyle S.: Ultrasonic diagnosis of altered fetal growth by use of a normal ultrasonic fetal weight curve. *Obstet. Gynecol.* 63:201–204, 1984.

Poll V., Kasby C.B.: An improved method of fetal weight estimation using ultrasound measurements of fetal abdominal circumference. *Br. J. Obstet. Gynaecol.* 86:922–928, 1979.

Rossavik I.K., Deter R.L.: The effect of abdominal profile shape changes on the estimation of fetal weight. *J. C. U.* 12:57–59, 1984.

Sabbagha R.E.: Intrauterine growth retardation, in Sabbagha R.E. (ed.): *Diagnostic Ultrasound Applied to Obstetrics and Gynecology*. New York, Harper & Row, pp. 103–110, 1980.

Sampson M.B., Thomason J.L., Kelly S.L., et al.: Prediction of intrauterine fetal weight using real-time ultrasound. *Am. J. Obstet. Gynecol.* 142:554–556, 1982.

Sarti D.A., Crandall B.F., Winter J., et al.: Correlation of biparietal and fetal body diameters: 12–26 weeks gestation. *A.J.R.* 137:87–91, 1981.

Shepard M.J., Richards V.A., Berkowitz R.L., et al.: An evaluation of two equations for predicting fetal weight by ultrasound. *Am. J. Obstet. Gynecol.* 142:47–54, 1982.

Tamura R.K., Sabbagha R.E.: Assessment of fetal weight, in Sabbagha R.E. (ed.): *Diagnostic Ultrasound Applied to Obstetrics and Gynecology*. New York, Harper & Row, pp. 93–102, 1980.

Thompson T.R., Manning F.A.: Estimation of volume and weight of the perinate: relationship to morphometric measurement by ultrasonography. *J. Ultrasound Med.* 2:113–116, 1983.

Wladimiroff J.W., Bloemsma C.A., Wallenburg H.C.S.: Ultrasonic assessment of fetal head and body sizes in relation to normal and retarded fetal growth. *Am. J. Obstet. Gynecol.* 131:857–860, 1978.

## Functional Evaluation of the Fetus

Bowie J.D., Clair M.R.: Fetal swallowing and regurgitation: observation of normal and abnormal activity. *Radiology* 144:877–878, 1982.

Fox H.E.: Fetal breathing, in Sabbagha R.E. (ed.): *Diagnostic Ultrasound Applied to Obstetrics and Gynecology.* New York, Harper & Row, pp. 199–209, 1980.

Gelman S.R., Wood S., Spellacy W.N., et al.: Fetal movements in response to sound stimulation. *Am. J. Obstet. Gynecol.* 143:484–485, 1982.

Manning F.A.: Monitoring fetal breathing using real-time ultrasound. *Hosp. Pract.* 19:72, 1979.

Manning F.A., Morrison I., Lange I.R., et al.: Antepartum determination of fetal health: composite biophysical profile scoring, Symposium on Fetal Monitoring. *Clin. Perinatol.* 9:285–296, 1982.

Manning F.A., Platt L.D., Sipos L.: Antepartum fetal evaluation: development of a fetal biophysical profile. *Am. J. Obstet. Gynecol.* 136:787–795, 1980.

Patrick J., Natale R., Richardson B.: Patterns of human fetal breathing activity at 34 to 35 weeks' gestational age. *Am. J. Obstet. Gynecol.* 132:507–513, 1978.

Picker R.H.: A scoring system for the morphological ultrasonic assessment of fetal well-being and maturation, in Lerski R.A., Morley P. (eds.): *Ultrasound '82.* Oxford, Pergamon Press Inc., 1983, pp. 597–601.

Platt L.D., Manning F.A.: A biophysical profile of the human fetus, in Sabbagha R.E. (ed.): *Diagnostic Ultrasound Applied to Obstetrics and Gynecology.* New York, Harper & Row, 1980, pp. 415–420.

Platt L.D., Manning F.A., Lemay M., et al.: Human fetal breathing: relationship to fetal condition. *Am. J. Obstet. Gynecol.* 132:514–518, 1978.

Rayburn W.F.: Antepartum fetal assessment. Monitoring fetal activity, Symposium on Fetal Monitoring. *Clin. Perinatol.* 9:231–252, 1982.

# CHAPTER 3

# Early Development

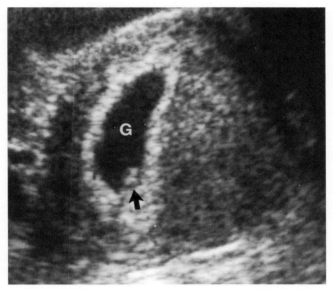

**Fig 3–1.**—Fetal pole. Seven-week intrauterine gestational sac *(G)* surrounded by a uniformly thick echogenic rind representing developing trophoblastic tissue. A 5- to 6-mm fetal "pole" is identified dependently *(arrow)*. The fetal pole or embryo as such can first be identified at approximately 6 weeks gestational age when it is approximately 4–5 mm in length. Early fetal cardiac activity has been identified between 41 and 43 days of gestation by documenting a persistent flicker of activity adjacent to the developing yolk sac. This is at a stage when identification of the actual embryo is most difficult. The developing embryo remains relatively shapeless with delineation of anatomic landmarks difficult until the 8th–9th week of gestational age.

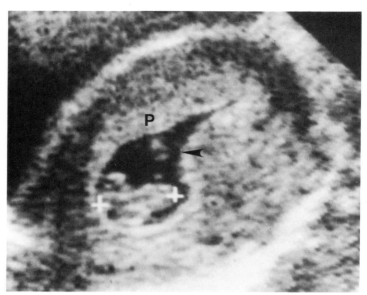

**Fig 3–2.**—Crown-rump length *(CRL).* Electronic calipers indicate a CRL of 1.9 cm corresponding to a gestational age of 8 weeks. The yolk sac *(arrowhead)* is noted anteriorly within the gestational sac. *P* = developing placenta. The CRL is the most accurate determination of gestational age obtainable throughout pregnancy, variously reported as being accurate to within plus or minus 3–6 days. The most accurate determinations are made at the 31- to 40-mm stage, which is between 10–11 weeks of gestational age. Earlier than 10 weeks, the CRL is shorter and therefore there is more measurement insensitivity. With gestational age beyond 12 weeks, increased fetal movement and flexibility makes accurate determination of the CRL more difficult.

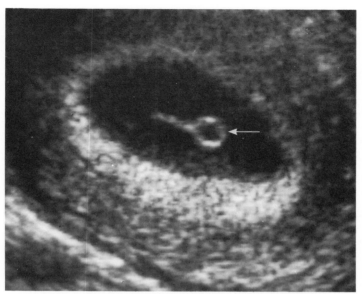

**Fig 3–3.**—Yolk sac *(arrow)* and adjacent amniotic membrane are apparent within the uterine cavity. The yolk sac is a spherical or ovoid, fluid-filled structure ranging in size from 2–7 mm, and lying external to the amniotic cavity. In some cases, only the brightly echogenic anterior and posterior walls are appreciated. It can be appreciated between 7–11 weeks in nearly all cases, and has been seen as early as 6 weeks plus 2 days or as late as 12 weeks plus 3 days. It is generally not appreciated after 11–12 weeks as the amniotic cavity enlarges to fill the uterine cavity, compressing the yolk sac against the uterine wall. There is a rough positive correlation between yolk sac size and crown-rump length. Conversely, a reduced size or absent yolk sac has been found in association with some congenital anomalies. It is important that the yolk sac is identified as a structure separate from the fetus so it is not inappropriately included in a crown-rump length determination.

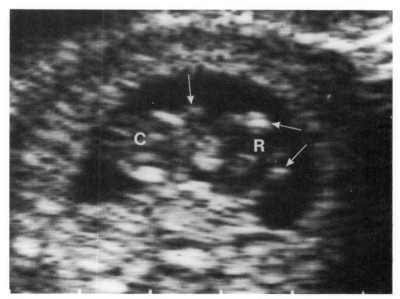

**Fig 3–4.**—Limb buds, coronal section, 9 weeks. Upper and lower extremity limb buds *(arrows)* can be identified. *C* = crown. *R* = rump.

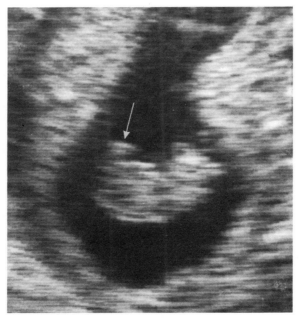

**Fig 3–5.**—Crown-rump length, limb bud, sagittal section, 9.5 weeks. Crown-rump length indicates a 9.5-week gestation. Lower extremity limb bud is identified *(arrow)*. More anatomic detail is becoming apparent at this stage of gestation.

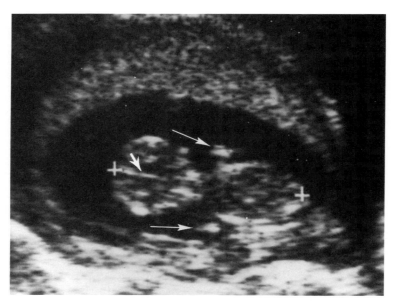

**Fig 3–6.**—Crown-rump length of 4.9 cm indicates a gestational age of 11.5 weeks. Coronal section delineates the interhemispheric fissure *(short arrow)* within the fetal skull, and the upper extremities *(long arrows)*. Lower extremities are out of the plane of section.

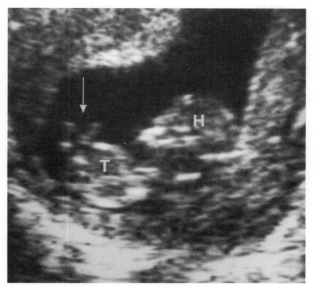

Fig 3–7.—Sagittal section, 11.5 weeks. Head (H) and trunk (T) are approximately equal in size in the first trimester. Longer lower extremities are now seen (arrow).

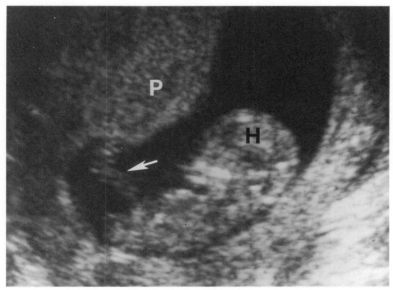

Fig 3–8.—Umbilical cord (arrow) is apparent, extending from the placenta (P) to the umbilical area in an 11.5-week fetus. H = head. The spiral appearance of the vessels within the cord is apparent even at this early stage.

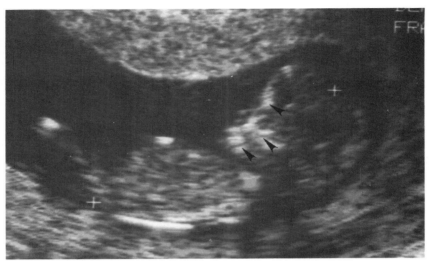

**Fig 3–9.**—Face, 11.5 weeks. Facial structures including the echogenic mandible, maxilla, and bony orbit *(arrowheads)* can be appreciated. A lower extremity is seen in extension. Electronic calipers may have slightly underestimated crown-rump length at the crown end.

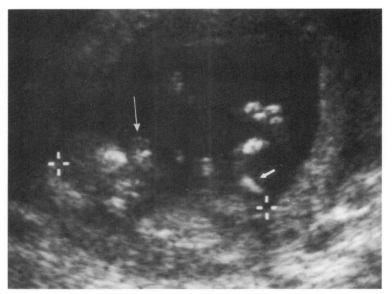

**Fig 3–10.**—Crown-rump length, 12 weeks. The fetus is in a supine position, with a crown-rump length by electronic calipers of 5.3 mm corresponding to a gestational age of 12 weeks. A fetal hand *(long arrow)* can be seen in front of the face; and several bones including the femur *(short arrow)* can be appreciated within the lower extremities. The accuracy of a crown-rump length diminishes from 12 weeks on due to increased fetal flexibility and motion. Furthermore, the bi-parietal diameter (BPD) may be difficult to obtain prior to 14 weeks gestational age, resulting in a relatively less accurate assignment of fetal age when scanning is performed between 12–14 weeks.

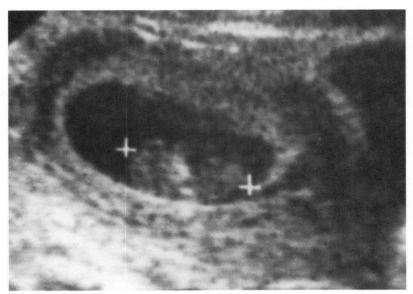

**Fig 3–11.**—Pitfall in CRL determination. The electronic calipers are incorrectly placed past both crown and rump, overestimating the CRL.

## REFERENCES

Cadkin A.V., McAlpin J.: Detection of fetal cardiac activity between 41 and 43 days of gestation. *J. Ultrasound Med.* 3:499–503, 1984.

Crooij M.J., Westhuis M., Schoemaker J., et al.: Ultrasonographic measurement of the yolk sac. *Br. J. Obstet. Gynaecol.* 89:931–934, 1982.

Drumm J.E., Clinch J., MacKenzie G.: The ultrasonic measurement of fetal crown-rump length as a method of assessing gestational age. *Br. J. Obstet. Gynaecol.* 83:417–421, 1979.

Fleischer A.C., James A.E. Jr., Davies J., et al.: Sonographic depiction of pregnancy during embryonic development, in Sanders R.C., James A.E. Jr. (eds.): *The Principles and Practice of Ultrasonography in Obstetrics and Gynecology.* New York, Appleton-Century-Crofts, 1985, pp. 61–75.

Lyons E.A., Levi C.S.: Ultrasound in the first trimester of pregnancy, in Callen P.W. (ed.): *Ultrasonography in Obstetrics and Gynecology.* Philadelphia, W.B. Saunders Co., 1983, pp. 1–19.

Mantoni M., Pedersen J.F.: Ultrasound visualization of the human yolk sac. *J. C. U.* 7:459–460, 1979.

Nelson L.H.: Comparison of methods for determining crown-rump measurement by real-time ultrasound. *J. C. U.* 9:67–70, 1981.

O'Brien G.D., Queenan J.T.: Dating gestation in the first 20 weeks, in Sanders R.C., James A.E. Jr. (eds.): *The Principles and Practice of Ultrasonography in Obstetrics and Gynecology.* New York, Appleton-Century-Crofts, 1985, pp. 141–146.

Pedersen J.F.: Fetal crown-rump length measurement by ultrasound in normal pregnancy. *Br. J. Obstet. Gynaecol.* 89:926–930, 1982.

Robinson H.P.: Sonar measurement of the fetal crown-rump length as a means of assessing maturity in the first trimester of pregnancy. *Br. Med. J.* 4:28–31, 1973.

Robinson H.P., Fleming J.E.E.: A critical evaluation of sonar "crown-rump length" measurements. *Br. J. Obstet. Gynaecol.* 82:702–710, 1975.

Sabbagha R.E., Kipper I.: The first trimester pregnancy, in Sabbagha R.E. (ed.): *Diagnostic Ultrasound Applied to Obstetrics and Gynecology.* New York, Harper & Row, 1980, pp. 59–67.

Sauerbrei E., Cooperberg P.L., Poland B.J.: Ultrasound demonstration of the normal fetal yolk sac. *J. C. U.* 8:217–220, 1980.

CHAPTER **4**

# Head and Neck

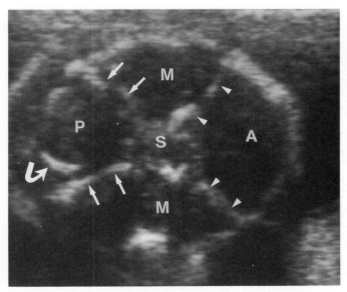

**Fig 4–1.**—Bony landmarks, base of skull, 23 weeks. Axial scan through the skull base shows the petrous pyramids *(arrows)* and sphenoid wings *(arrowheads)* delineating the posterior *(P),* middle *(M),* and anterior *(A)* cranial fossae. *Curved arrow* indicates margin of foramen magnum. *S* = region of sella turcica.

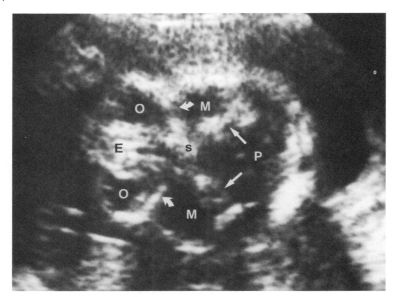

**Fig 4–2.**—Bony landmarks, base of skull, 20 weeks. Axial section through skull base at lower level than in Figure 4–1. Petrous pyramids *(straight arrows)* and sphenoid wings *(curved arrows)* separate posterior *(P)* and middle *(M)* fossae and the bony orbits *(O)*. Ethmoid bones *(E)* separate the orbits. *S* = region of sella turcica.

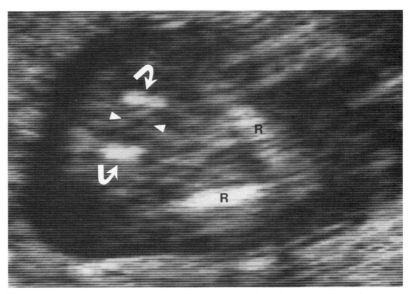

**Fig 4–3.**—Foramen magnum, 15 weeks. Axial section at the very base of the skull demonstrates bright echogenic foci posteriorly delineating the margins of the foramen magnum *(curved arrows)*. A central, circular echogenic structure with a hypoechoic center represents the upper cervical spinal cord *(arrowheads)*. Rami of the mandible are seen anteriorly *(R)*.

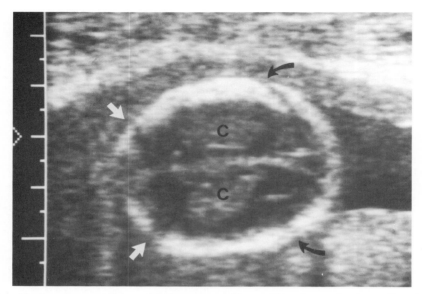

**Fig 4–4.**—Skull sutures. High axial image. Coronal *(curved arrows)* and lambdoid *(straight arrows)* sutures can be appreciated as disconti-nuities within the calvarium. Prominent, echo-genic choroid plexus *(C)* is seen within the lateral ventricles.

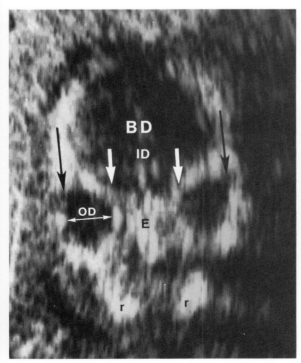

**Fig 4–5.**—Face, 15.5 weeks. Coronal image of the face demonstrates the rami of the mandible *(r)*, ethmoid/nasal bone complex *(E)*, and bony orbits. Various ocular measurements that can be derived include the binocular distance *(BD, black arrows)*, the interorbital distance *(ID, white arrows)*, and the ocular diameter *(OD)*. Such measurements have been correlated with BPD determinations to assess for various bony orbit abnormalities, including hypotelorism/hypertelorism, and microophthalmia. For accurate measurement of ocular dimensions, a symmetrical image of the orbits must be obtained.

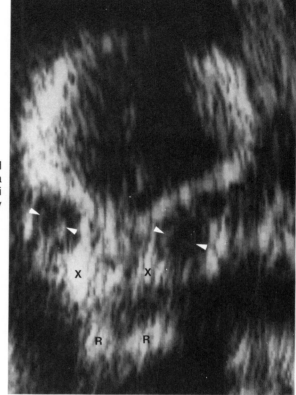

**Fig 4–6.**—Facial bones, 15.5 weeks. Coronal scan anterior to Figure 4–5 delineates the maxilla *(X),* and more medial parts of the mandibular rami *(R).* Lenses *(arrowheads)* are noted centrally within the bony orbits.

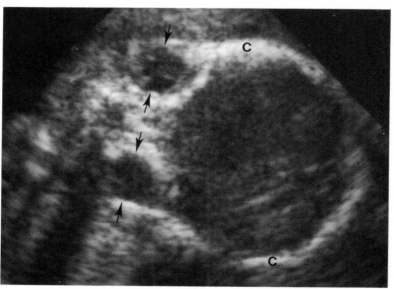

**Fig 4–7.**—Fetal orbits, 20 weeks. Angled axial image demonstrates a larger cross-section of the fetal calvarium *(C)* and less of the face than Figure 4–5. This image through the bony orbits *(arrows)* is obtained by starting with a normal BPD image and angling caudally at the anterior aspect of the skull until the orbits are imaged. As axial resolution is superior to lateral resolution, this technique will assure optimal imaging of the medial and lateral orbital walls for accurate measurements.

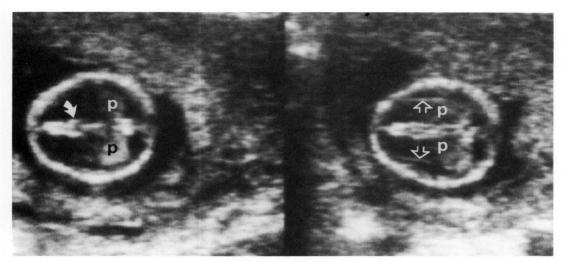

**Fig 4–8.**—Early biparietal diameter *(BPD),* 13 weeks, axial sections. **Left,** while the thalami may be difficult to identify at this age, the cavum septum pellucidum can usually be seen as bright parallel echoes *(curved arrow),* and an ovoid calvarial image at this level is a good approximation for BPD determination. **Right,** lateral walls of the frontal horns and bodies of the lateral ventricles are seen bilaterally *(open arrows).* Note the very thin mantle of hypoechoic cerebral parenchyma at this early gestational age. The very prominent choroid plexus *(p)* is imaged within the lateral ventricles.

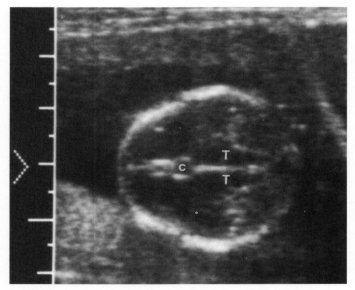

**Fig 4–9.**—Early biparietal diameter, 14 weeks. The hypoechoic cerebral peduncle/thalami complex *(T)* and the cavum septum pellucidum *(c)* confirm an appropriate axial section for a BPD measurement of 28 mm. Early in gestation, intracranial landmarks may be difficult to distinguish. When the hypoechoic thalamic region or the bright walls of the cavum septum pellucidum cannot be identified, the prominent choroid plexus may serve as a guideline for obtaining an axial section. Coronal sutures are seen as anterolateral calvarial discontinuities.

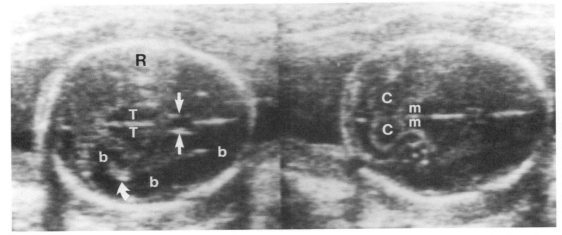

**Fig 4–10.**—BPD, 20 weeks. **Left,** axial scan through the hypoechoic thalami *(T)* and the cavum septum pellucidum *(straight arrows)* more anteriorly is appropriate for a BPD determination. Note the hypoechoic cerebral parenchyma *(b)* surrounding echogenic choroid plexus *(curved arrow)* within the trigone of the lateral ventricle. This is only appreciated on the far side of the brain, as the reverberations *(R)* obscure the finding in the near field. **Right,** scan at a lower level demonstrates the hypoechoic cerebral peduncles/midbrain *(m)* and the cerebellar hemispheres *(C),* the latter surrounded by cerebrospinal fluid within the cisterna magna and adjacent subarachnoid spaces. While the **left** image is considered optimal for BPD determination, the **right** image measures only slightly smaller. Hence, when the thalami are not well delineated, a BPD through the peduncles/midbrain may suffice.

**Fig 4–11.**—Biparietal diameter, anatomic landmarks, 31 weeks. Axial section at the level of the hypoechoic, heart-shaped thalami *(T).* The third ventricle, bordered by echogenic margins *(short straight arrow),* is between the thalami. The cavum septum pellucidum is a larger, midline fluid-filled structure *(large solid curved arrows)* that lies between the frontal horns *(open curved arrows* indicate lateral walls). It extends superiorly and posteriorly to a variable degree between the bodies of the lateral ventricles as the cavum vergae. The anterior aspect of the echogenic falx cerebri/interhemispheric fissure is identified with a *short curved arrow.* These structures should be identified in the midline, with strong calvarial echoes bilaterally. Electronic calipers ($\pm$) indicate appropriate measurement points for a biparietal diameter determination extending from the outer margin of the near calvarial echo to the inner margin of the far calvarial echo. Measurements can also be made from inner-to-outer margins and from mid-to-mid calvarial echo. *A* = anterior.

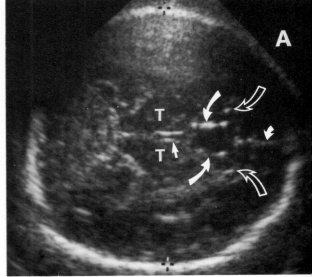

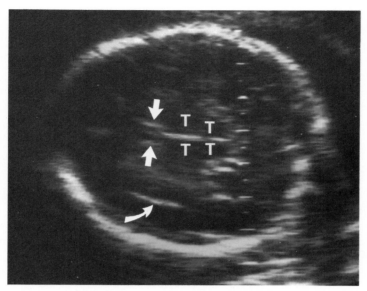

**Fig 4–12.**—Biparietal determination, 25 weeks. Even with a suboptimal examination due to equipment or maternal obesity, one can usually delineate cerebral structures sufficiently to obtain an adequate BPD. In this case, the thalami *(T)* and the cavum septum pellucidum *(straight arrows)* are just well enough differentiated from adjacent structures, so that an appropriate section for BPD determination could be imaged. *Curved arrow* indicates the sylvian fissure/insula surrounded by normal echopenic brain.

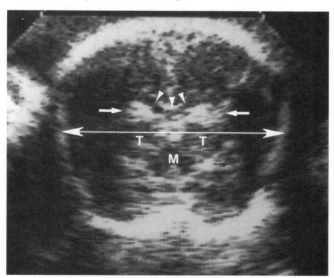

**Fig 4–13.**—Coronal biparietal diameter determination. Thalami *(T)* and midbrain *(M)* are hypoechoic structures lying inferior to the echogenic choroid plexus within the lateral and third ventricles *(arrows)*. The *two-ended arrow* indicates the approximate level through the thalami for measuring the BPD. It is apparent that an axial section obtained above this level would yield a larger BPD measurement; however, as anatomic landmarks are less reproducible, the level through the thalami has become standard. The hypoechoic corpus callosum has a wide "V" configuration superior to the ventricles *(arrowheads)*. Coronal determination of the biparietal diameter is not as accurate as axial determination, as anatomic landmarks are less reproducible, and lateral rather than axial resolution is employed for identifying calvarial landmarks. It may be used as an approximation, however, in cases where an accurate axial measurement is not possible, as long as the image is symmetrical and traverses the thalami.

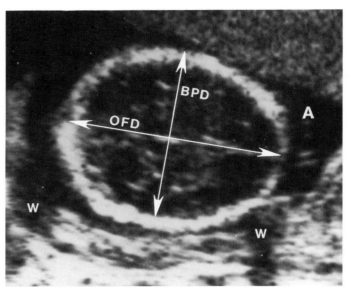

**Fig 4–14.**—Cephalic index, 18 weeks. The cephalic index is defined as the ratio of the biparietal diameter *(BPD)* to the occipitofrontal diameter *(OFD)* measured from mid to mid calvarial echo. The normal ratio is .74–.83, with deviations from this suggesting an abnormality of calvarial shape. If the ratio is low, the BPD should not be used as a predictor of gestational age as it may be abnormally low. A head circumference measurement is then preferable. It may be difficult to image the entire calvarium simultaneously due to refraction at the lateral scan margins, seen here in occipital and frontal regions with associated shadowing *(W). A* = anterior.

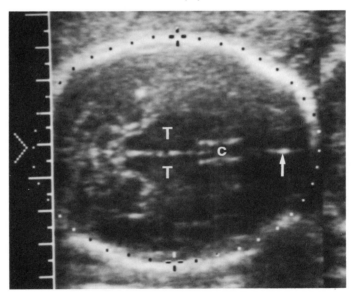

**Fig 4–15.**—Head circumference (HC), 27 weeks. Axial section through the thalami *(T),* cavum septum pellucidum *(c),* and interhemispheric fissure *(arrow)* is appropriate for BPD determination. Electronic calipers (+) demarcate the BPD and the HC (indicated by the *ovoid series of dots).* HC is useful in gestation age determination when the cephalic index (Fig 4–14) is low, and in consort with other parameters for evaluation of intrauterine growth retardation.

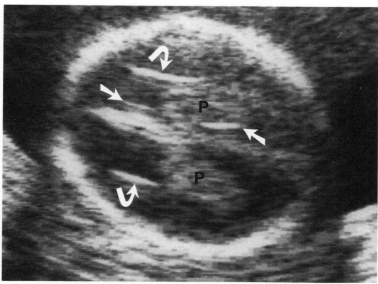

**Fig 4–16.**—Lateral ventricle, frontal horn, 16 weeks. Axial section cephalad to the level for determining biparietal diameter shows large echogenic choroid plexus *(P)*. The echogenic lateral margins of both frontal horns *(curved arrows),* and medial walls of the body and frontal horn on one side *(straight arrows)* are seen. A complete cranial survey involves more than obtaining a BPD. In the exclusion of hydrocephalus, scanning must be performed above the level for a biparietal diameter determination so as to visualize the ventricles. Normal measurements relating various ventricular landmarks to brain or calvarial dimensions (i.e., lateral ventricular width/hemispheric width) have been defined to aid in the diagnosis of ventriculomegaly.

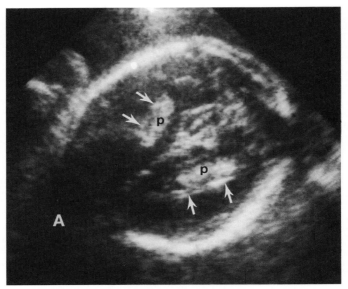

**Fig 4–17.**—Lateral ventricle, body, 23 weeks. Axial image through the bodies of the lateral ventricles reveals echogenic choroid plexus *(p)* flush with the lateral wall of the ventricles *(arrows)*. The echogenic ventricular walls are difficult to image unless they are perpendicular to the scan plane. Note the orientation of the ventricles, spreading apart posteriorly to accommodate for the structures of the posterior fossa. *A* = Anterior.

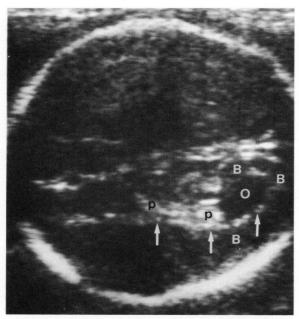

**Fig 4–18.**—Lateral ventricle, occipital horn. Axial section shows choroid plexus *(p)* filling the body of the lateral ventricle (*arrows* indicate lateral margin). The anechoic occipital horn *(O)*, centrally located within the hypoechoic cerebral parenchyma *(B)*, extends back towards the midline.

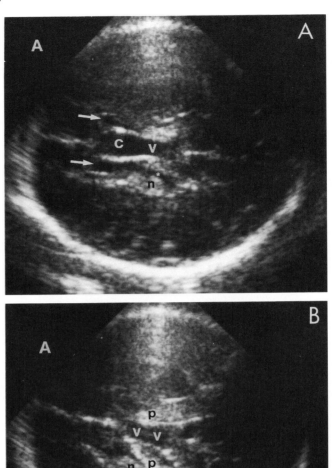

**Fig 4–19.**—Lateral ventricles, cavum septum pellucidum, cavum vergae. Axial scans above the level of the thalami are necessary to image the bodies of the lateral ventricles. *A* = anterior. **A,** prominent fluid-filled cavum septum pellucidum *(C)* lies between the frontal horns *(arrows)* anteriorly and extends posterior to the foramen of Monro as the cavum vergae *(V)*. The moderately echogenic head of the caudate nucleus *(n)* is seen adjacent to the floor of the lateral ventricle *(∗)*. **B,** axial scan above **A.** The very echogenic choroid plexus *(p)* is now seen within the bodies of the lateral ventricles, separated by a short extension of the cavum vergae *(V)*. Note the angled orientation of the lateral ventricle being more medial anteriorly and lateral posteriorly. *n* = caudate nucleus.

*Continued.*

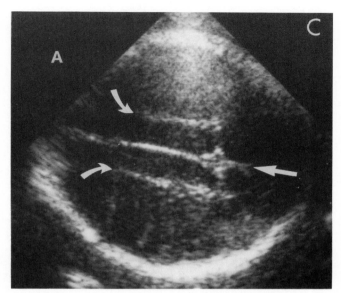

**Fig 4–19 Cont.**—**C,** a high axial section delineates the interhemispheric fissure *(straight arrow)* paralleled by two echogenic linear structures *(curved arrows)*. While these latter structures may represent the superolateral walls of the lateral ventricles, linear echoes can be imaged well cephalad to the level of the lateral ventricles (**D** and **E**). As such they would not be affected by ventricular enlargement and hence not useful in the diagnosis of hydrocephaly.

*Continued.*

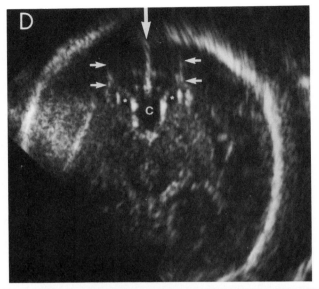

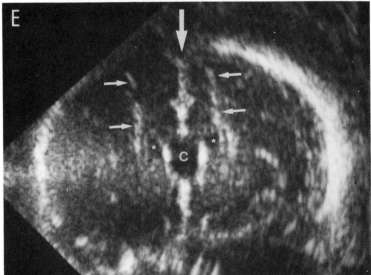

**Fig 4–19 *Cont.*—D** and **E,** coronal images through the frontal horns *(∗)* and the cavum septum pellucidum *(C)*. The echogenic midline interhemispheric fissure is indicated with an arrow. The parallel, paramidline, echogenic linear structures imaged in **C** are seen to extend from approximately the superolateral aspect of the lateral ventricles well into brain substance beyond the location of the ventricles *(arrows).* The anatomic explanation for this finding is unclear. However, it appears that the three parallel echogenic line configurations on high axial images **(C)** do not necessarily represent ventricular margins.

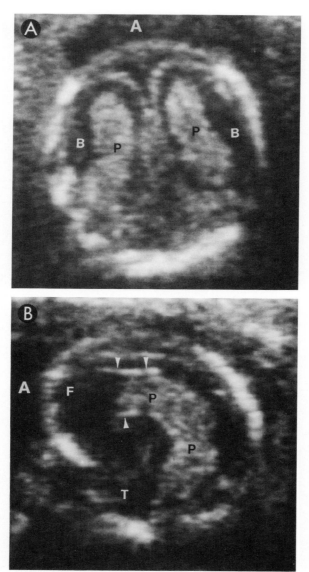

**Fig 4–20.**—Choroid plexus, 15 weeks. Angled coronal **(A)** and parasagittal **(B)** scans through the fetal calvarium demonstrate the normal extensive echogenic choroid plexus **(P)** filling the body and trigone of the lateral ventricle at this gestational age. The choroid plexus is very prominent in the late first and early second trimester during its glycogen-rich phase. Superior and inferior ventricular margins are delineated in **B** by *arrowheads*. The relatively large size of the lateral ventricles, and the smaller rim of hypoechoic cerebrum *(B)* is clearly depicted in **A.** *F* = frontal lobe. *T* = temporal lobe. *A* = anterior.

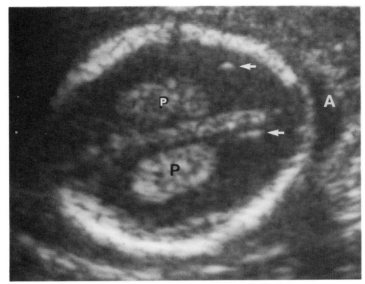

**Fig 4–21.**—Choroid plexus, 16 weeks. High axial section demonstrates prominent hyperechoic choroid plexus *(P)* filling the body of the lateral ventricle. The choroid plexus does not extend into the frontal horn. *Arrows* indicate lateral wall of near ventricle and medial wall of far ventricle. *A* = anterior.

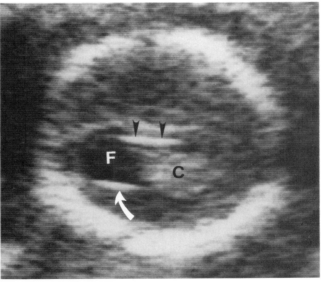

**Fig 4–22.**—Choroid plexus, ventricular wall relationship. High axial section delineates prominent choroid plexus *(C)* within the body of the lateral ventricle, extending from the medial *(arrowheads)* to the lateral *(curved arrow)* walls of the ventricle. With normal ventricular size, the choroid plexus will extend from the medial to the lateral wall of the body of the ventricle (the choroid plexus does not extend into the frontal horn *[F]*). With hydrocephalus, a diminutive choroid plexus is imaged that will not oppose both ventricular margins.

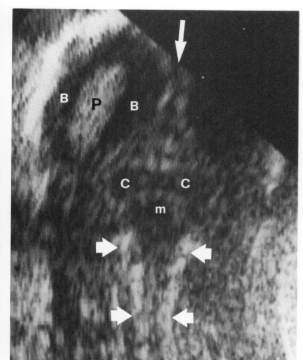

**Fig 4–23.**—Choroid plexus, 17 weeks. Oblique coronal image through the upper cervical spine *(short arrows)* and brain. The echogenic, bulky choroid plexus *(P)* is seen filling the lateral ventricle and surrounded by hypoechoic brain *(B)*. *Long arrow* indicates midline. The normal widening of the upper cervical spine is appreciated just caudad to the posterior fossa where one sees the cerebellar hemispheres *(C)* and cisterna magna *(m)*.

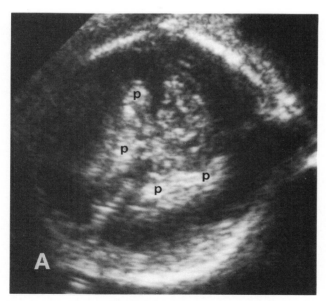

**Fig 4–24.**—Choroid plexus, 23 weeks. Axial section through the ventricles reveals the choroid plexus *(p)* as considerably smaller than in the early second trimester; however, it still fills the entire width of the bodies of the lateral ventricles as the hypoechoic cerebrum grows.

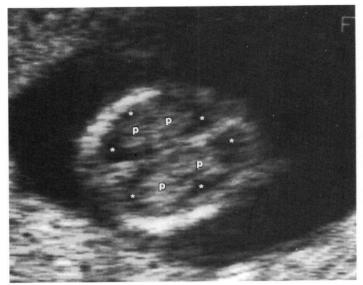

**Fig 4–25.**—Cerebral cortex, 13 weeks. High axial image demonstrates the very large, echogenic choroid plexus *(p)* within the lateral ventricles which nearly fill both cerebral hemispheres. Such a thin, hypoechoic cerebral mantle *(*)* is normal at this stage prior to significant brain growth.

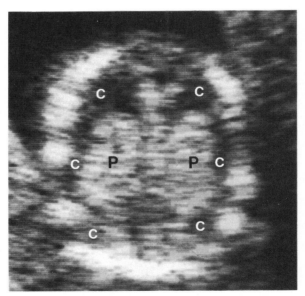

**Fig 4–26.**—Cerebral cortex, 15 weeks. High axial image demonstrates extensive echogenic choroid plexus *(P)* filling the lateral ventricles, surrounded in turn by the normal, relatively thin, echopenic developing cerebrum *(C)*.

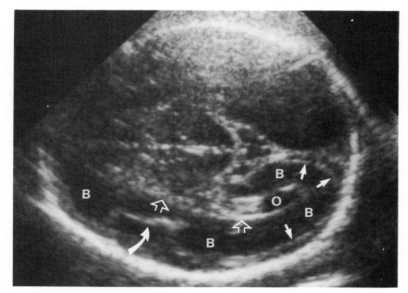

**Fig 4–27.**—Cerebral parenchyma, sylvian fissure/insula, 26 weeks. Normal cerebral parenchyma *(B)* remains hypoechoic throughout pregnancy. The echogenic margins of the occipital cortex *(closed straight arrows),* surrounding the occipital horn of the lateral ventricle *(O),* are appreciated posteriorly. Between this cortical margin and the calvarium and falx lies the hypoechoic subarachnoid space. A linear echogenic structure which is the sylvian fissure/insula *(curved arrow)* should not be mistaken for the lateral wall of the ventricle which is more medially located *(open arrows).* The ventricle and the echogenic choroid plexus within the body of the lateral ventricle are considerably smaller than earlier in the second trimester.

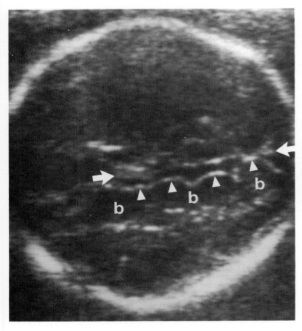

**Fig 4–28.**—Cerebral gyri. A higher axial section shows the echogenic curvilinear margins of the cerebral gyri *(arrowheads)* overlying echopenic brain *(b). Arrows* indicate falx/interhemispheric fissure, separated from the gyri by subarachnoid fluid.

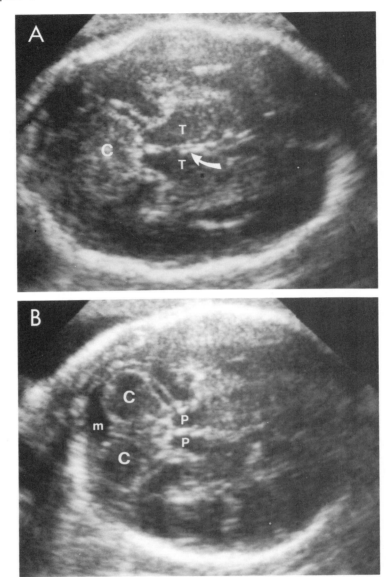

**Fig 4–29.**—Thalamus, midbrain, 26 weeks. Axial sections, 26 weeks. **A,** hypoechoic heart-shaped thalami *(T)* surround the slit-like third ventricle *(arrow).* The cephalic portion of the cerebellum *(C)* is just posterior to the thalami. **B,** a lower section shows the smaller, slightly more posterior, hypoechoic cerebral peduncles/midbrain *(P),* anterior to the well-defined cerebellar hemispheres *(C). m* = cisterna magna.

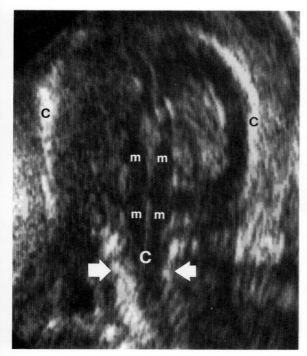

**Fig 4–30.**—Brain stem, cervical cord, 16 weeks. Angled coronal scan through the calvarium *(black C)* and upper cervical spine *(arrows)* shows the hypoechoic brain stem *(m)* in contiguity with the upper cervical spinal cord *(white C)*.

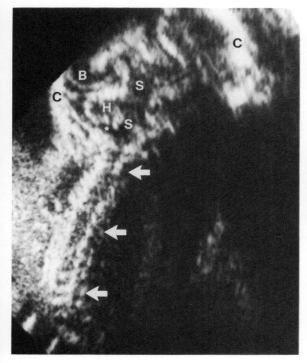

**Fig 4–31.**—Brain stem, posterior fossa, 25 weeks. Sagittal scan through the cervicothoracic spine *(arrows)* and the fetal calvarium *(C)*. Intracranially, the hypoechoic brain stem *(S)*, cerebellum *(H)*, cisterna magna *(\*)*, and occipital cortex *(B)* are identified.

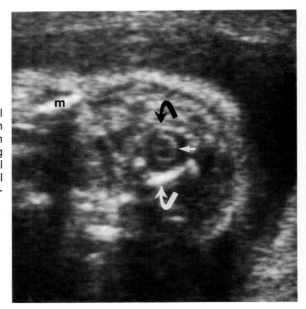

**Fig 4–32.**—Brain stem, upper cervical spinal cord. Angled axial image through the foramen magnum *(curved arrows)* delineates the brain stem/cervical cord as a thin echogenic ring around a hypoechoic core, with small central echogenic focus representing the central canal *(straight arrow). m* = mandible with distal shadowing.

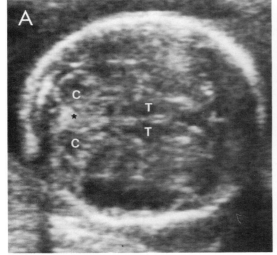

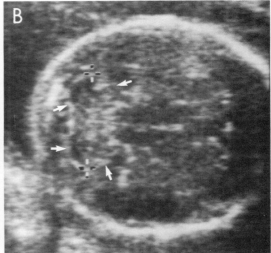

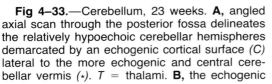

**Fig 4–33.**—Cerebellum, 23 weeks. **A,** angled axial scan through the posterior fossa delineates the relatively hypoechoic cerebellar hemispheres demarcated by an echogenic cortical surface *(C)* lateral to the more echogenic and central cerebellar vermis *(∗). T* = thalami. **B,** the echogenic margins of the hemispheres can be appreciated *(arrows),* and electronic calipers *( + )* mark appropriate points for determining cerebellar width. Cerebellar measurements correlate closely with BPD, and may be of value in evaluating various posterior fossa abnormalities.

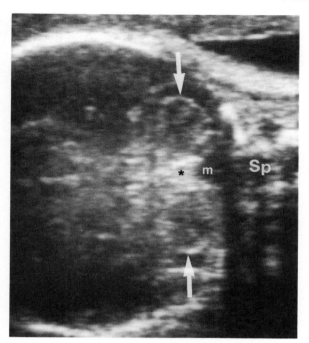

**Fig 4–34.**—Cerebellum, 27 weeks. Coronal image through the posterior fossa delineates the echogenic midline cerebellar vermis *(\*)* and the hypoechoic lateral cerebellar hemispheres with their echogenic margins *(arrows)*. The cisterna magna *(m)* is a fluid-filled structure in the midline posteroinferiorly. *Sp* = upper cervical spine.

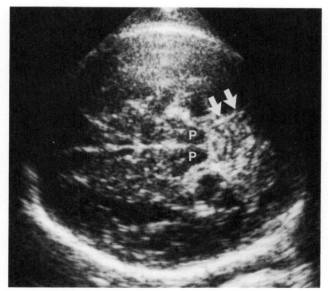

**Fig 4–35.**—Cerebellar folia, 32 weeks. Axial section demonstrates the cerebellar folia as several curvilinear echogenic lines *(arrows)* over the surface of the hemispheres. *P* = peduncles.

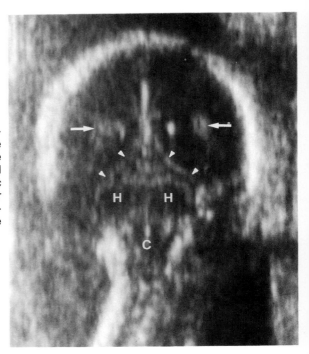

**Fig 4–36.**—Tentorium, 18 weeks. Angled coronal image through the posterior fossa shows the cerebellar hemispheres *(H)*, upper cervical spine and cord *(C)*, and choroid plexus within the lateral ventricles *(arrows)* surrounded by hypoechoic cerebrum. The echogenic margins of the superior part of the tentorium *(arrowheads)* can be appreciated between the cerebral hemispheres and the cerebellum.

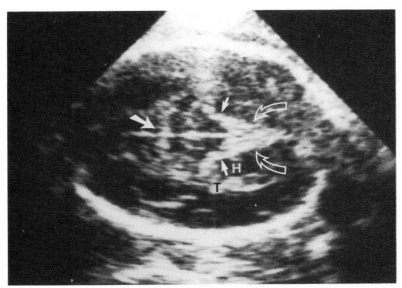

**Fig 4–37.**—Cisterns. Axial scan. An echogenic arrowhead configuration is formed by the quadrigeminal plate cistern *(curved arrows)* and the ambient cisterns *(straight arrows)* which demarcate the posterolateral margins of the midbrain and communicate anteriorly with the echogenic interpeduncular cistern *(slanted arrow)*. H = hypoechoic hippocampus, located between the ambient cistern and the trigone of the lateral ventricle *(T)*.

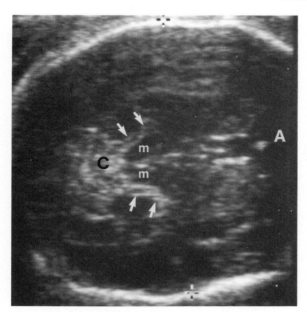

**Fig 4–38.**—Cisterns, 30 weeks. Axial section through the midbrain *(m)*. The echogenic quadrigeminal plate cistern *(C)* is less pronounced than in Figure 4–37. The thinner, echogenic ambient cisterns *(arrows)* extend anterolaterally around the midbrain. *A* = anterior.

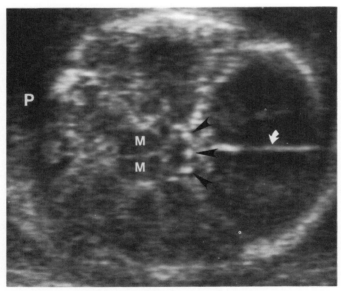

**Fig 4–39.**—Cerebral vessels, 25 weeks. Axial section through the midbrain *(M)* near the skull base. Several bright punctate echoes anterior to the brain stem represent vascular structures in the region of the circle of Willis *(arrowheads)*. The basilar artery can frequently be seen on real-time as a brightly pulsating echo just anterior to the brain stem. *Curved arrow* indicates interhemispheric fissure between the frontal lobes. *P* = posterior.

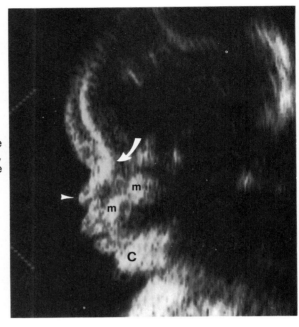

**Fig 4–40.**—Face, profile. Parasagittal image close to the midline shows the mandible/chin (C), lips, nose (arrowhead), and medial aspect of the bony orbit (curved arrow). m = maxilla.

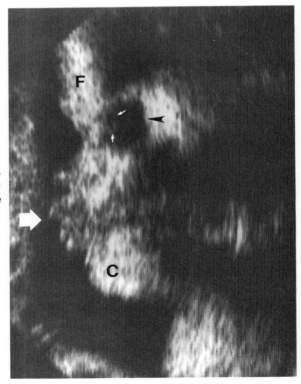

**Fig 4–41.**—Face, profile, 28 weeks. Parasagittal scan demonstrates the bony orbit (arrowhead) and lens anteriorly (small arrows), frontal bone (F), nose, lips (wide arrow), and chin (C).

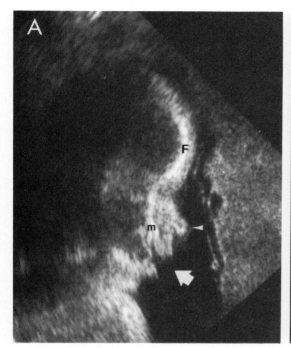

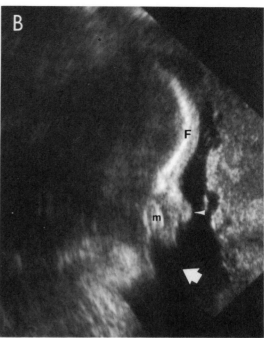

**Fig 4–42.**—Face, profile. Mouth opening. Midline sagittal scans through the face demonstrate a partially open (**A**) and a wide open (**B**) mouth *(arrow). Arrowhead* indicates nose. *F* = frontal bone. *m* = maxilla.

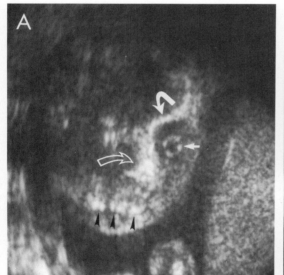

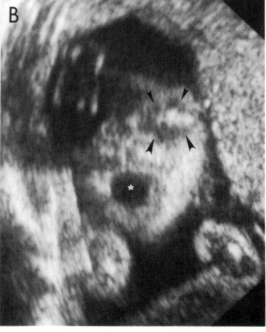

**Fig 4–43.**—Face, eyelids, lens. Oblique coronal images. **A,** the bony orbit *(closed curved arrow),* nasal bones *(open arrow),* and several tooth buds *(arrowheads)* can be appreciated. The lens of the eye is a central echogenic ring within the bony orbit *(straight arrow).* **B,** a more anterior section shows the closed eyelids *(arrowheads)* and an open mouth/lips *(∗).*

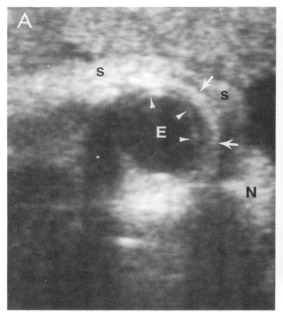

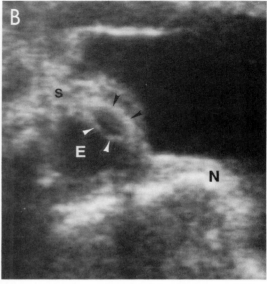

**Fig 4–44.**—Eyelid, globe, lens. Angled axial sections through the left eye *(E)*. *N* = region of nose, *S* = soft tissues of cheek. **A,** thin, curvilinear echogenic line within the orbit is the margin of the globe *(arrowheads)*. The thicker eyelid immediately overlaps the globe *(arrows)*. **B,** oblique section through the globe cephalad to **A** shows the margins of the lens as a lenticular echogenic structure *(arrowheads)* anteriorly within the globe.

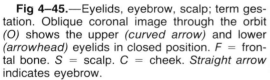

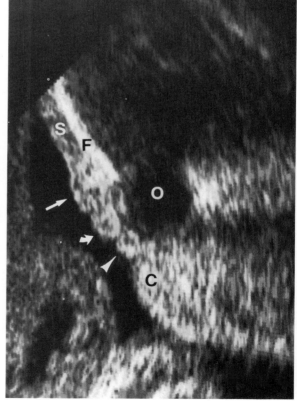

**Fig 4–45.**—Eyelids, eyebrow, scalp; term gestation. Oblique coronal image through the orbit *(O)* shows the upper *(curved arrow)* and lower *(arrowhead)* eyelids in closed position. *F* = frontal bone. *S* = scalp. *C* = cheek. *Straight arrow* indicates eyebrow.

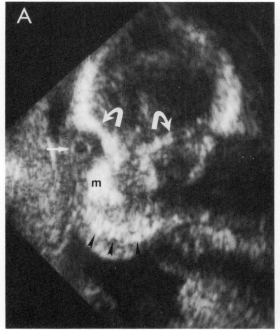

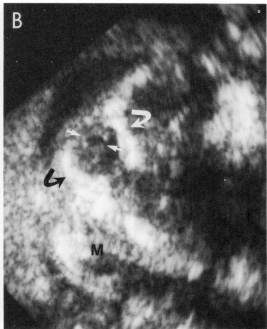

**Fig 4–46.**—Fetal eye movement, 20 weeks. **A,** coronal section through the face delineates the bony orbits *(curved arrows),* right maxilla *(m),* and multiple echogenic tooth buds *(arrowheads).* The lens of the right eye, identified as an echogenic circle *(straight arrow),* is in neutral position within the orbit. **B,** motion of the eye is noted as the lens is now "looking" upward toward the orbital roof *(straight arrows)* with an asymmetrical position within the bony orbit *(curved arrows). M* = mouth.

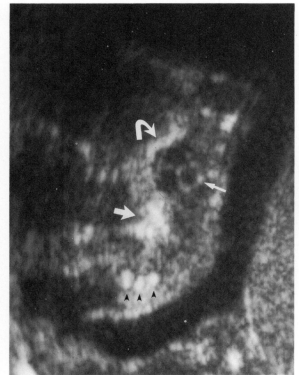

**Fig 4–47.**—Face, toothbuds, 22 weeks. Oblique coronal image through the face reveals the circular, echogenic lens *(thin arrow)* within the bony orbit *(curved arrow),* nasal bones *(wide arrow),* and three toothbuds *(arrowheads).* Teeth begin to ossify in the early second trimester.

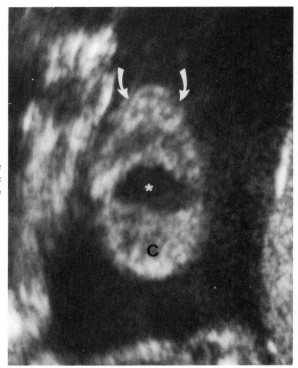

**Fig 4–48.**—Mouth, 22 weeks. Coronal image demonstrates an open mouth containing amniotic fluid *(*)*, the soft tissues of the chin *(C)*, and the very tip of the nose *(arrows)*.

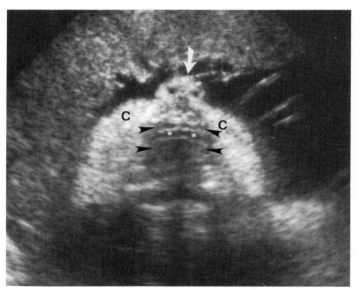

**Fig 4–49.**—Cheeks, lips, nose. Coronal image through the lower face demonstrates the hypoechoic lips *(arrowheads)*, slightly open with intervening amniotic fluid *(*)*. Plump soft tissues of the cheeks *(C)* are lateral to the nose *(arrow)*.

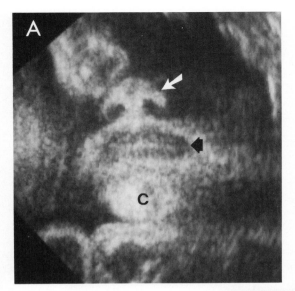

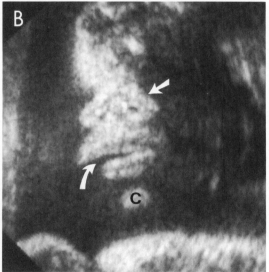

**Fig 4–50.**—Nose, mouth, lips, chin. Angled coronal images through the anterior lower face show the nose with amniotic fluid in the nares *(slanted arrows)*. C = chin. **A,** mouth is closed with the hypoechoic lips slightly opposed *(black arrow)*. Such an image is useful in screening for a cleft lip. **B,** mouth is slightly open with the lips separated *(curved arrow)*.

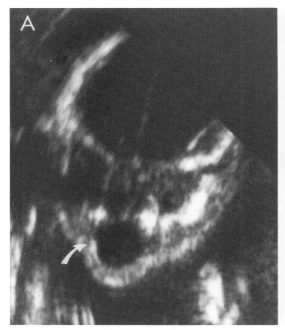 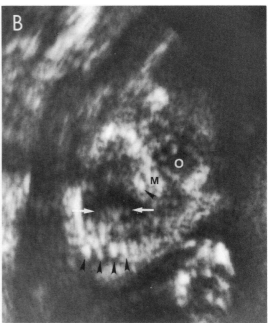

**Fig 4–51.**—Mouth, tongue, toothbuds. **A,** coronal image through the face shows a wide open mouth *(arrow).* **B,** a more posterior section shows the mouth partially open with amniotic fluid around the tongue *(arrows). Arrowheads* indicate toothbuds. *M* = maxilla. *O* = orbit.

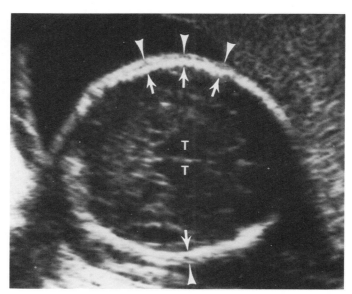

**Fig 4–52.**—Scalp, 29 weeks. Axial section through the thalami *(T)* for biparietal diameter measurement. The less echogenic scalp of several millimeters thickness *(arrowheads)* should be differentiated from the more echogenic underlying calvarium *(arrows),* so as not to overestimate the biparietal diameter.

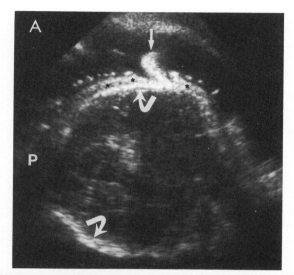

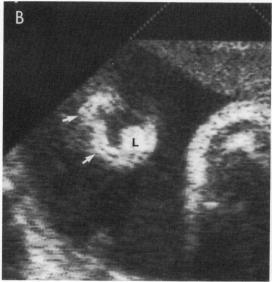

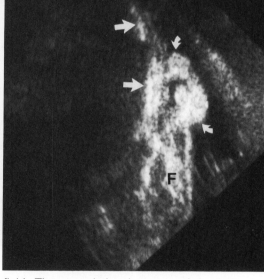

**Fig 4–53.**—Ear, hair. **A,** axial section. The ear *(straight arrow)* is directed posteriorly *(P)* from its attachment at the scalp *(*)*. Multiple punctate echogenic foci adjacent to the scalp both anterior and posterior to the ear represent fetal hair. *Curved arrows* indicate calvarium. **B,** sagittal/tangential image of the ear surrounded by amniotic fluid. The convolutional pattern of the helix *(arrows)* and the larger, inferiorly positioned lobule *(L)* are appreciated. **C,** roughly coronal scan through the ear showing the pinna projecting laterally *(curved arrows)* between the calvarium *(straight arrows)* and posterior face *(F)*.

**Fig 4–54.**—Craniocervical soft tissue, 25 weeks. Coronal image through the cervical region demonstrates the proximal humerus *(H)* surrounded by soft tissues of the shoulder girdle, the bony calvarium *(C),* and the cervical and upper thoracic spine *(P).* Note the normal prominence of the soft tissues in the craniocervical region *(S)* which should not be mistaken for a soft tissue mass. Scan transversely where possible to document symmetry between sides and to define the normal gentle convexity of outer body margins at this level.

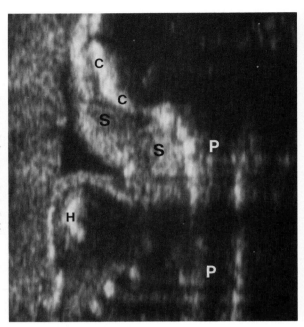

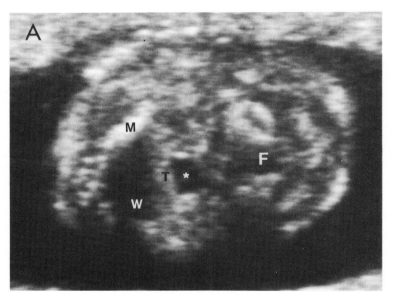

**Fig 4–55.**—Hypopharynx, tongue, trachea, 20 weeks. **A,** angled axial scan near the craniocervical junction delineates the mandible *(M)* with distal shadowing *(W),* anteriorly. The hypopharynx is a fluid-filled region *(\*)* posterior to the tongue *(T)* which is partially shadowed by the mandible. Tongue movement, presumably associated with swallowing, can frequently be observed. *F* = foramen magnum.

*Continued.*

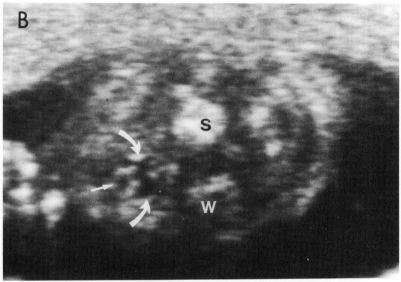

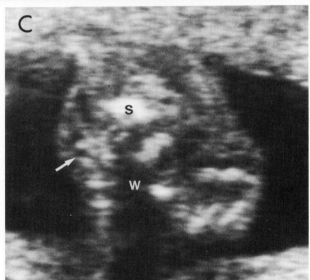

**Fig 4–55 Cont.**—**B,** axial section through the upper cervical region shows the trachea *(straight arrow)* splitting off anteriorly from the hypopharynx. The upper esophagus/piriform sinuses *(curved arrows)* are seen posteriorly. *S* = cervical spine with distal shadowing *(W)*. **C,** angled axial scan through the lower cervical spine demonstrates the fluid-filled trachea anteriorly within the neck *(arrow)*. *S* = spine with distal shadowing *(W)*.

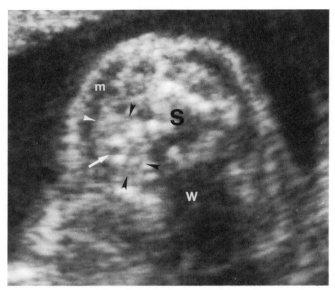

**Fig 4–56.**—Thyroid, trachea, strap muscles. Axial section through the mid-neck delineates the fluid-filled trachea *(arrow)* lying anteromedially to the mildly echogenic lobes of the thyroid *(arrow-heads)*. S = cervical spine with distal shadowing *(W)*. m = hypoechoic strap muscles of anterolateral neck.

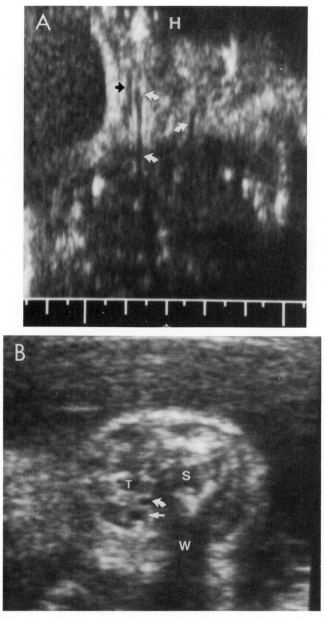

**Fig 4–57.**—Carotid artery, jugular vein. Coronal **(A)** and axial **(B)** images show the carotid artery *(curved arrows)* medially, and jugular vein *(straight arrows)* laterally within the neck. *T* = midline, fluid-filled trachea. *S* = cervical spine with distal shadowing *(W)*. *H* = head.

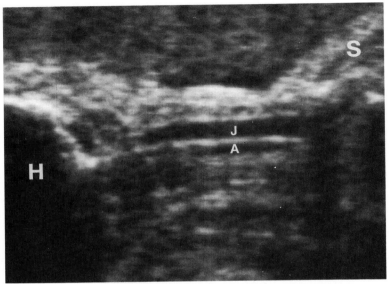

**Fig 4–58.**—Carotid artery, jugular vein, 31 weeks. Angled coronal image through the neck delineates the wider, tubular jugular vein *(J),* superficial to the thinner carotid artery *(A). H =* head. *S =* shoulder.

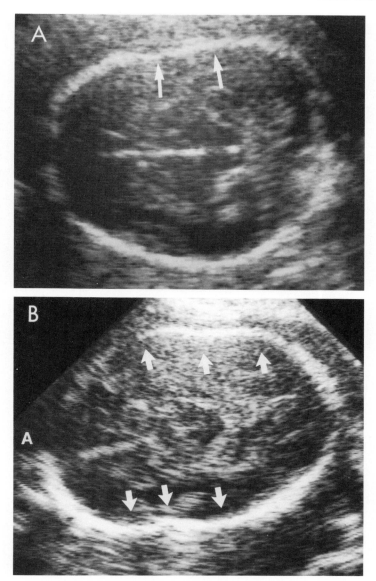

**Fig 4–59.**—Pitfall in BPD determination. Pressure deformity. **A,** axial section through the calvarium for BPD determination at 19 weeks demonstrates a mild anterior contour deformity *(arrows)* secondary to pressure applied during scanning. **B,** both near and far calvarial contour changes *(arrows)* exist secondary to pressure applied during scanning. *A* = anterior. Such alterations in calvarial contour can result in erroneous BPD determinations.

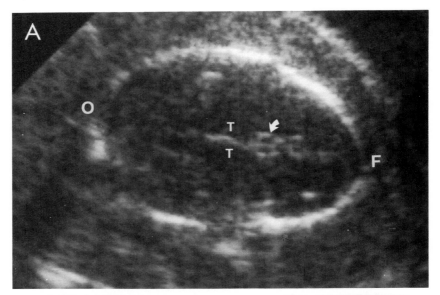

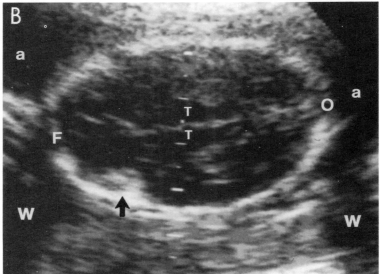

**Fig 4–60.**—Pitfall in BPD determination. Dolichocephaly. **A,** dolichocephalic calvarial configuration secondary to ruptured membranes, 16 weeks. Axial section through thalami *(T)* and cavum septum pellucidum *(arrow)*. A dolichocephalic configuration with a narrow width (BPD) and increased length (OFD = occipitofrontal diameter) has resulted from oligohydramnios. The cephalic index (CI = BPD/OFD) of .67 is low, suggesting that a gestational age based on BPD may be artifactually low. *F* = frontal. *O* = occiput. **B,** axial image reveals a long, thin (dolichocephalic) configuration to the calvarium at the level of the thalami *(T)*. The cephalic index is correspondingly low at .64 (normal = .74–.83). This scan is mildly obliqued and a roof of one orbit can be seen *(arrow)*. *a* = amniotic fluid. *O* = occiput. *F* = frontal. *W* = refractive shadowing from the portions of the laterally positioned calvarium within the image. When the CI is low, measurement of long bone length or head circumference would be preferable to BPD for gestational age determination. In general, fetal evaluation is considerably more difficult when oligohydramnios is present, as fetal structures are compressed together and into unusual locations.

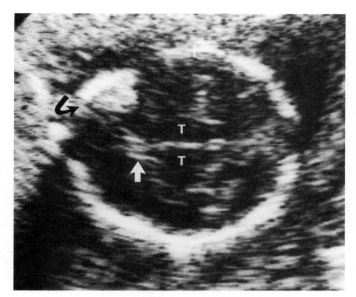

**Fig 4–61.**—Pitfall in BPD determination, oblique scan, 16 weeks. Angled axial scan through the thalami *(T)* and cavum septum pellucidum *(straight arrow)*. A technically suboptimal image for BPD determination is indicated by the asymmetry of the scan which is too low on one side, including a plaque-like echogenic structure which is the orbital roof *(curved arrow)*.

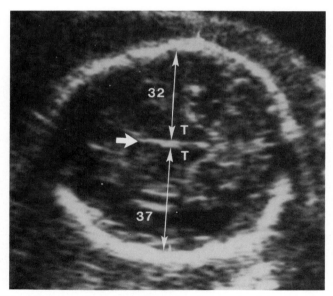

**Fig 4–62.**—Pitfall in biparietal diameter measurement, asymmetrical midline echo, 27 weeks. While the thalami *(T)* are reasonably well imaged, the midline echo *(arrow)* is considerably closer to the near calvarial echo *(32* mm) than the distal echo *(37* mm). Inaccurate biparietal diameter measurements may result from such asymmetrical scans.

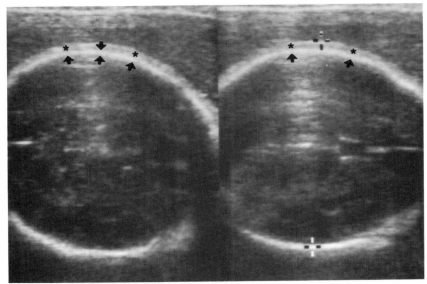

**Fig 4–63.**—Pitfall in BPD determination, scalp, 29 weeks. Without **(Left)** and with **(Right)** electronic calipers *( + )*. It is important when electronic calipers are used to verify placement at the appropriate landmarks for measurement. The near caliper is actually placed on the outer skin margin of the scalp *(∗)*, a midlevel band of echoes surrounding the echogenic calvarium *(arrows)*. The far caliper marker is placed midway within the calvarial echo rather than at the inner margin. In this instance, the electronic caliper measurement was 80.1 mm (31 weeks) versus a hand measurement of 74 mm (<29 weeks). Such measurement errors can lead to significant discrepancies in assigning gestational age, particularly in the third trimester when head growth is slowest.

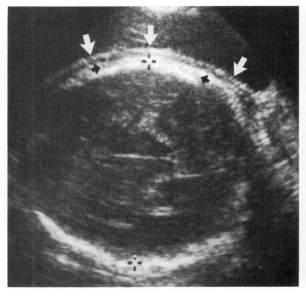

**Fig 4–64.**—Pitfall in BPD or scalp thickness determination, maternal bladder wall, 33 weeks. On axial section, electronic calipers *( + )* mark the outer margin of the near calvarial echo and the inner margin of the far calvarial echo appropriately for BPD determination. The low level echoes external to the proximal calvarial echo represent the fetal scalp *(black arrows)*, demarcated by the echogenic skin surface. A third curvilinear echogenic line *(white arrows)* is the posterior wall of the maternal bladder which frequently is closely positioned over the head in the third trimester. The bladder wall should not be mistaken for the outer calvarial margin, leading to an erroneously large BPD determination. Additionally, the bladder wall could be taken to be the skin margin, which might suggest fetal hydrops.

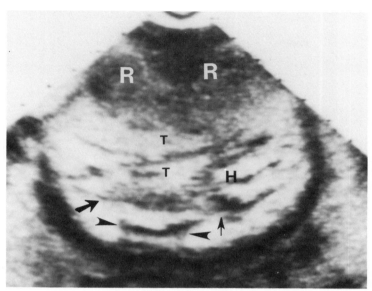

**Fig 4–65.**—Pitfall, normal echopenic brain mistaken for hydrocephalus, brain cysts, fluid collections, 27 weeks. Axial section shows central, hypoechoic, heart-shaped thalami *(T)*. The near side of the brain is obscured by echogenic reverberation artifact *(R)*. Within the dependent portion of brain, multiple normally hypoechoic areas of cerebral parenchyma are not infrequently mistaken for hydrocephalus, extra-axial fluid collections, etc. Identification of interposed normal landmarks such as the trigone of the lateral ventricle *(straight arrow)* lateral to the hippocampus *(H)*, the lateral margin of the frontal horn *(slanted arrow),* and the sylvian fissure/insula *(arrowheads)* will help delineate the remaining hypoechoic areas as normal cerebrum. Objective standards exist for measuring displacements of the above landmarks with ventriculomegaly. Subjectively, with hydrocephalus the various echogenic interfaces normally within brain are not seen. Only the echogenic choroid plexus, diminutive in size, will be seen internally as the fluid-filled ventricles expand to reach the midline and compress brain laterally.

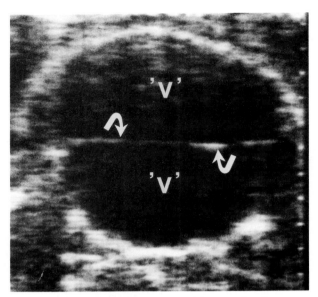

**Fig 4–66.**—Pitfall, hydrocephalus secondary to inadequate gain, 35 weeks. With greater calvarial ossification in the third trimester, insufficient gain may cause poor penetration and visualization of intracranial structures. In this case, only the highly echogenic interhemispheric fissure *(ar-rows)* is seen leading to a mistaken impression of grossly dilated, fluid-filled ventricles *('V')*. Increasing the gain and scanning in different planes should allow for adequate visualization of intracranial structures for the exclusion of hydrocephalus.

## REFERENCES

Aantaa K., Forss M.: Growth of the fetal biparietal diameter in different types of pregnancies. *Radiology* 137:167–169, 1980.

Birnholz J.C.: The fetal external ear. *Radiology* 147:819–821, 1983.

Buttery B.W.: Occipitofrontal-biparietal diameter ratio. An ultrasonic parameter for the antenatal evaluation of Down's syndrome. *Med. J. Aust.* 2:662–664, 1979.

Case K.J., Hirsch J., Case M.J.: Simulation of significant pathology by normal hypoechoic white matter in cranial ultrasound. *J. C. U.* 11:281–285, 1983.

Chervenak F.A., Berkowitz R.L., Romero R., et al.: The diagnosis of fetal hydrocephalus. *Am. J. Obstet. Gynecol.* 147:703–716, 1983.

Chinn D.H., Callen P.W., Filly R.A.: The lateral cerebral ventricle in early second trimester. *Radiology* 148:529–531, 1983.

Christ J.E., Meininger M.G.: Ultrasound diagnosis of cleft lip and cleft palate before birth. *Plast. Reconstr. Surg.* 68:854–859, 1981.

Crade M., Patel J., McQuown D.: Sonographic imaging of the glycogen stage of the fetal choroid plexus. *A.J.R.* 137:489–491, 1981.

Davies P., Richardson R.E.: Dynamic fetal cephalometry. *Br. J. Obstet. Gynaecol.* 86:765–772, 1979.

de Elejalde M.M., Elejalde B.R.: Visualization of the fetal face by ultrasound. *J. Craniofac. Genet. Dev. Biol.* 4:251–257, 1984.

Denkhaus H., Winsberg F.: Ultrasonic measurement of the fetal ventricular system. *Radiology* 131:781–787, 1979.

Deter R.L., Harrist R.B., Hadlock F.P., et al.: Fetal head and abdominal circumferences: I. Evaluation of measurement errors. *J. C. U.* 10:357–363, 1982.

Fiske C.E., Filly R.A.: Ultrasound evaluation of the normal and abnormal fetal neural axis, in Callen P.W. (ed.): *Ultrasonography in Obstetrics and Gynecology.* Philadelphia, W.B. Saunders Co., 1983, pp. 97–112.

Fleischer A.C., Entman S.S.: The importance of the scan plane in fetal ventricular size assessment. *J. C. U.* 11:229–230, 1983.

Ford K.B., McGahan J.P.: Cephalic index: its possible use as a predictor of impending fetal demise. *Radiology* 143:517–518, 1982.

Hadlock F.P., Deter R.L., Carpenter R.J., et al.: Estimating fetal age: effect of head shape on BPD. *A.J.R.* 137:83–85, 1981.

Hadlock F.P., Deter R.L., Harrist R.B., et al.: Fetal head circumference: relation to menstrual age. *A.J.R.* 138:649–653, 1982.

Hadlock F.P., Deter R.L., Harrist R.B., et al.: Fetal biparietal diameter: rational choice of plane of section for sonographic measurement. *A.J.R.* 138:871–874, 1982.

Hadlock F.P., Deter R.L., Park S.K.: Real-time sonography: ventricular and vascular anatomy of the fetal brain in utero. *A.J.R.* 136:133–137, 1981.

Hadlock F.P., Harrist R.B., Shah Y., et al.: The femur length/head circumference relation in obstetric sonography. *J. Ultrasound Med.* 3:439–442, 1984.

Hughey M.J.: Fetal cephalometry, in Sabbagha R.E. (ed.): *Diagnostic Ultrasound Applied to Obstetrics and Gynecology.* New York, Harper & Row, 1980, pp. 69–78.

Jeanty P., Cantraine F., Cousaert E., et al.: The binocular distance: a new way to estimate fetal age. *J. Ultrasound Med.* 3:241–243, 1984.

Jeanty P., Chervenak F.A., Romero R., et al.: The sylvian fissure: a commonly mislabeled cranial landmark. *J. Ultrasound Med.* 3:15–18, 1984.

Jeanty P., Dramaix-Wilmet M., Van Gansbeke D., et al.: Fetal ocular biometry by ultrasound. *Radiology* 143:513–516, 1982.

Johnson M.L., Dunne M.G., Mack L.A., et al.: Evaluation of fetal intracranial anatomy by static and real-time ultrasound. *J. C. U.* 8:311–318, 1980.

Kasby C.B., Poll V.: The breech head and its ultrasound significance. *Br. J. Obstet. Gynaecol.* 89:106–110, 1982.

Kurtz A.B., Wapner R.J., Kurtz R.J., et al.: Analysis of biparietal diameter as an accurate indicator of gestational age. *J. C. U.* 8:319–326, 1980.

Laing F.C., Stamler C.E., Jeffrey R.B.: Ultrasonography of the fetal subarachnoid space. *J. Ultrasound Med.* 2:29–32, 1983.

Leveno K.J., Santos-Ramos R., Duenhoelter J.H., et al.: Sonar cephalometry in twin pregnancy: discordancy of the biparietal diameter after 28 weeks' gestation. *Am. J. Obstet. Gynecol.* 138:615–619, 1980.

Mayden K.L., Tortora M., Berkowitz R.L., et al.: Orbital diameters: a new parameter for prenatal diagnosis and dating. *Am. J. Obstet. Gynecol.* 144:289–297, 1982.

McGahan J.P., Phillips H.E.: Ultrasonic evaluation of the size of the trigone of the fetal ventricle. *J. Ultrasound Med.* 2:315–319, 1983.

McGahan J.P., Phillips H.E., Ellis W.G.: The fetal hippocampus. *Radiology* 147:201–203, 1983.

O'Brien W.F., Coddington C.C., Cefalo R.C.: Serial ultrasonographic biparietal diameters for prediction of estimated date of confinement. *Am. J. Obstet. Gynecol.* 138:467–468, 1980.

Ott W.J.: The use of ultrasonic fetal head circumference for predicting expected date of confinement. *J. C. U.* 12:411–415, 1984.

Sabbagha R.E.: Biparietal diameter and gestational age, in Sabbagha A.E. (ed.): *Diagnostic Ultrasound Applied to Obstetrics and Gynecology.* New York, Harper & Row, 1980, pp. 79–91.

Sabbagha R.E., Barton F.B., Barton B.A.: Sonar biparietal diameter: I. Analysis of percentile growth differences in two normal populations using same methodology. *Am. J. Obstet. Gynecol.* 126:479–484, 1976.

Sabbagha R.E., Barton B.A., Barton F.B., et al.: Sonar biparietal diameter: II. Predictive of three fetal growth patterns leading to a closer assessment of gestational age and neonatal weight. *Am. J. Obstet. Gynecol.* 126:485–490, 1976.

Sabbagha R.E., Hughey M., Depp R.: Growth adjusted sonographic age: a simplified method. *Obstet. Gynecol.* 51:383–386, 1978.

Smazal S.F. Jr., Weisman L.E., Hopper K.D., et al.: Comparative analysis of ultrasonographic methods of gestational age assessment. *J. Ultrasound Med.* 2:147–150, 1983.

Wolfson R.N., Zador I.E., Halvorsen P., et al.: Biparietal diameter in premature rupture of membranes: errors in estimating gestational age. *J. C. U.* 11:371–374, 1983.

# CHAPTER 5

# Spine

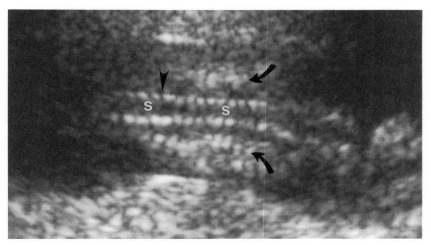

**Fig 5–1.**—Early spine delineation, 11.5 weeks. High resolution coronal image through the thoracolumbar spine *(S)* reveals individual ossification centers of the posterior lamina. Normal mild widening of the thoracolumbar junction is seen *(arrowhead).* Portions of several ribs *(arrows)* are noted.

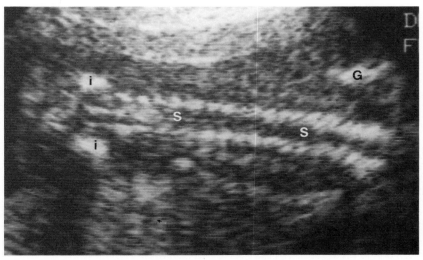

**Fig 5–2.**—Thoracolumbar spine, 15.5 weeks. Coronal image of the entire thoracolumbar spine *(S)* from the level of the shoulder girdle *(G)* to the iliac crests *(i).* While individual ossification centers are not clearly resolved throughout, the normal essentially parallel configuration is maintained.

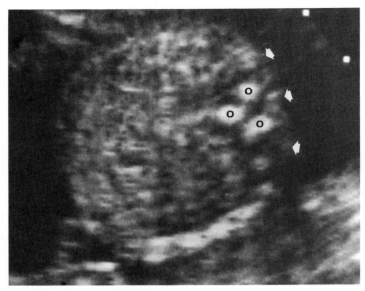

**Fig 5–3.**—Ossification centers, 17 weeks. A transverse section shows the three typical ossification centers *(O)* in the spine (lumbar illustrated), appropriately spaced in a tight triangular configuration. The anterior center is the developing vertebral body while the two posterior centers are the lamina. The posterior soft tissues are also evaluated and noted to be symmetrical and only as thick as normal muscle, with the skin surface smoothly convex *(arrows),* excluding a protruding midline mass.

$\longrightarrow$

**Fig 5–4.**—Sequential coronal images, complete spine, 22 weeks. Imaging in a coronal plane is a sensitive means for detecting a small widening in the posterior elements of the spine. Equal portions of the fetal body should be imaged on both sides of the spine to assure a correct coronal plane through the posterior ossification centers. Only early in gestation can one obtain a near-complete spine on a single image as the fetus tends to become curled in position in the second trimester, necessitating sequential coronal scans. **A,** within the lumbosacral spine, ossification centers of the posterior lamina *(long arrows)* are seen laterally, while ossification centers of several vertebral bodies are central *(short arrows).* It is difficult to image all three ossification centers in a single plane since they are in a triangular configuration. The slight smooth widening between the posterior lamina at the thoracolumbar junction is a normal finding. *C* = iliac crests. Roughly coronal images through the thoracic **(B)** and the cervicothoracic **(C)** spine delineate the normal parallel configuration of the posterior ossification centers with a normal mild widening in the upper cervical region *(∗).* *H* = head.

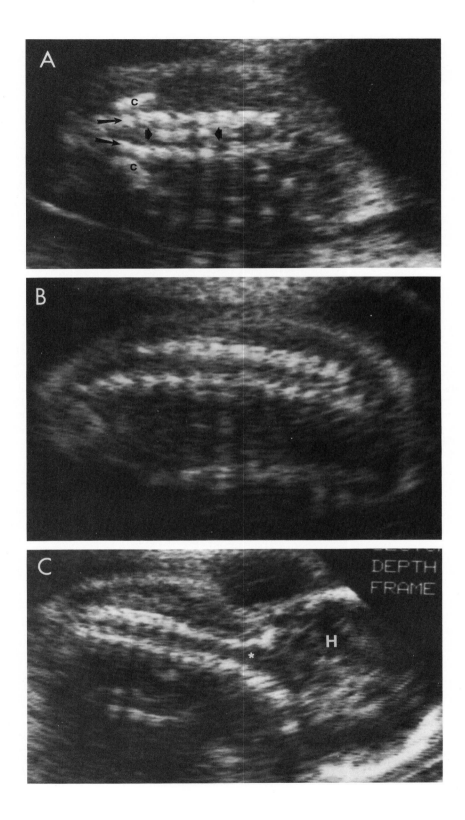

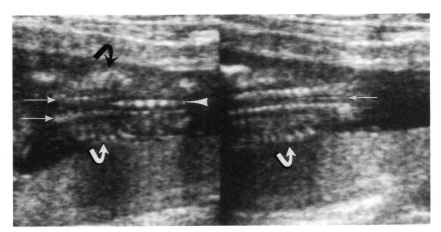

**Fig 5–5.**—Vertebra body ossification center versus spinal cord. Coronal images through the thoracolumbar spine at two depths differentiate the echoes of the vertebral body ossification centers from that of the spinal cord. The **left,** more anterior image, demonstrates the faint parallel echogenic ossification centers of the posterior lamina *(straight arrows).* In the lumbar region, the segmented hyperechoic central echoes represent the ossification centers of the vertebral body *(arrowhead).* The **right,** more posterior image, shows the parallel posterior ossification centers to better advantage. A thin, contiguous, and echogenic central line represents the central canal of the spinal cord *(straight arrow).* Multiple ribs can be seen *(curved arrows),* especially in the more anterior **left** image.

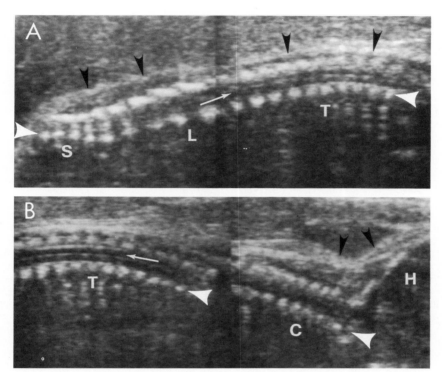

**Fig 5–6.**—Complete spine, 32 weeks. **A** and **B,** composite linear array images show the entire spine in the sagittal plane. *S* = sacral, *L* = lumbar, *T* = thoracic, *C* = cervical. The posterior row of ossification centers are posterior lamina on one side, while the anterior ossification centers are the vertebral bodies *(white arrowheads)*. Such longitudinal images can be used for orientation and assessing gross integrity of the spine. However, coronal scans simultaneously imaging both posterior elements are more sensitive for detecting subtle widening. The spinal cord can be seen within the spinal canal at several levels as echogenic lines representing the wall and/or central canal surrounded by hypoechoic neural tissue *(arrows)*. The normal prominence of the soft tissues posteriorly in the craniocervical and lumbosacral regions can be appreciated as the widened hypoechoic space between the posterior ossification centers and the skin *(black arrowheads)*. *H* = head. *Continued.*

→

**Fig 5–6** *Cont.*—**C–E,** sequential transverse images document the appearance of the spine and adjacent musculature. Such scanning from the occiput to the tip of the coccyx in the transverse plane is probably the most sensitive technique for discerning the presence of spinal defects. Transverse images also can be more routinely obtained than coronal images when the fetal spine is dependent or excessively tortuous. **C, left,** in the mid-cervical spine *(C),* the posterior lamina *(arrows)* are seen as linear rather than focal ossification centers at this more advanced gestational age. The hypoechoic posterior musculature is quite prominent in the neck *(arrowheads).* **C, right,** in the upper thoracic spine *(UT)* posterior laminae are again noted to be more linear than punctate *(arrows).* The scapulae *(s)* are seen within the hypoechoic musculature of the upper back/shoulder girdle *(m). Arrowheads* indicate ribs. **D, left,** in the lower thoracic spine *(LT),* the compact triangular configuration of the ossification centers is seen *(arrow).* The paraspinal musculature *(arrowheads)* is relatively thin at this point. *r* = ribs. **D, right,** in the upper lumbar spine *(UL),* the three echogenic ossification centers are well seen, and the paraspinal musculature remains relatively thin. The hypoechoic spinal cord *(arrow)* can be seen centrally within the spinal canal. **E, left,** hypoechoic paraspinal musculature *(m)* again becomes very prominent around the lower lumbar spine *(LL).* As at other levels within the spine, the normal posterior lamina ossification centers *(l)* are as close to each other as they are to the vertebral body ossification center *(b).* This relationship is important in excluding spina bifida. **E, right,** in the sacral spine *(S),* the paraspinal musculature remains prominent, although reduced in overall bulk. Three spinal ossification centers are still noted. When imaging the spine transversely, it is important to note not only the tight triangular configuration of the ossification centers with a smooth transition from level to level, but also to inspect the posterior skin surface to confirm a continuous smooth convex contour. The normal, broadly spaced, hypoechoic musculature should not be confused with a myelomeningocele which has a point of attachment centrally over the posterior aspect of the spine.

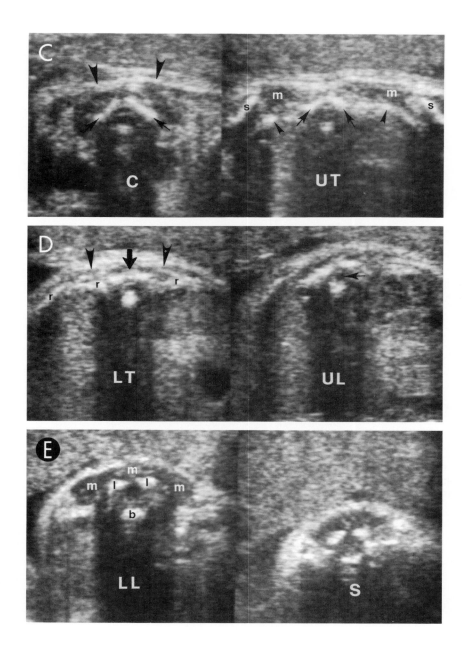

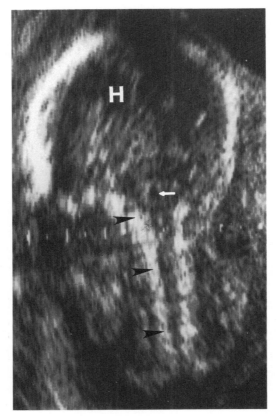

**Fig 5–7.**—Cervical spine, normal widening. Coronal image through the cervical spine *(arrowheads)* and head *(H)* at 20 weeks demonstrates normal widening of the upper cervical spine. The fourth ventricle *(arrow)* can be appreciated surrounded by the hypoechoic cerebellar hemispheres.

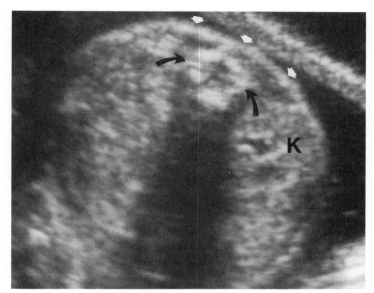

**Fig 5–8.**—Increasing spinal ossification. Transverse section through the upper lumbar spine at 28 weeks. Increasing ossification has led to a more ring-like configuration *(black arrows)* versus the earlier three punctate echo pattern. The posterior skin surface is intact, of uniform thickness, smooth, and gently convex *(white arrows)*. K = kidney.

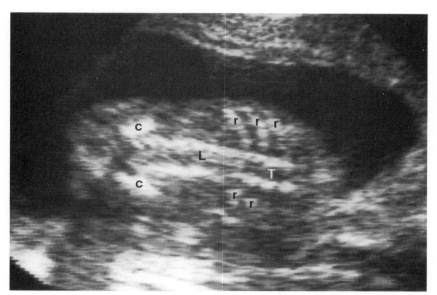

**Fig 5–9.**—Thoracolumbar spine, relation to ribs, sacroiliac joints. Coronal image through the lumbar *(L)* and lower thoracic *(T)* spine does not resolve individual ossification centers; however, spinal widening may still be excluded. Several posterior lower ribs *(r)* can be seen adjacent to the thoracic spine. The region of the sacroiliac (SI) joint is noted between the iliac crests *(c)* and the spine.

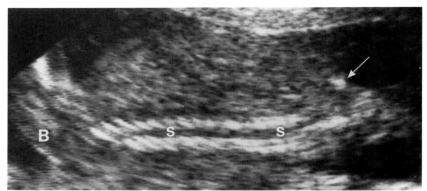

**Fig 5–10.**—Potential pitfalls of spine exam in supine fetus, 16 weeks. The spine may be difficult or impossible to image in coronal section with this fetal lie. While parallel ossification centers may be imaged, they usually represent the anteriorly positioned vertebral body and one side of the posterior lamina. This image would be insensitive for detecting spina bifida which is manifest as a widening between the posterior lamina. With such a fetal lie, transverse images must be relied on to detect splaying of the posterior lamina. There may also be some difficulty in identifying associated soft tissue masses projecting posteriorly from the spine due to penetration and focal depth considerations. Additionally, in this position the back is usually in contact with the myometrium rather than fluid, reducing natural contrast. *S* = spine. *B* = buttock. *Arrow* indicates cross-section of clavicle.

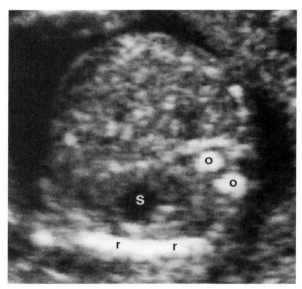

**Fig 5–11.**—Pitfall, transverse spine imaging. Oblique transverse scan through high lumbar spine at 18 weeks gestational age. The angled nature of the scan is apparent as only two spine ossification centers *(o)* are well identified. In addition, a long segment of rib *(r)* is identified on only the left side of the abdomen. *S* = stomach. For an accurate examination to detect widening of the spine, scanning must define a true transverse plane with the posterior ossification centers imaged simultaneously.

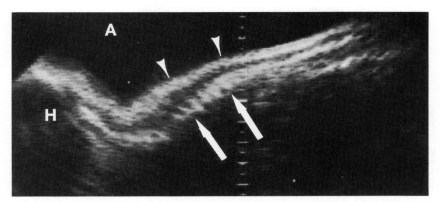

**Fig 5–12.**—Pitfall, longitudinal spine imaging. Longitudinal image through the cervicothoracic spine demonstrates the segmented nature usually apparent from vertebral ossification centers *(arrows)*. The parallel echogenic structure *(arrowheads)* is not another row of ossification centers but rather the skin margin which is hyperechogenic due to enhanced sound transmission through the adjacent amniotic fluid *(A)*. *H* = head.

REFERENCES

Filly R.A., Golbus M.S.: Ultrasonography of the normal and pathologic fetal skeleton, Symposium on Ultrasonography in Obstetrics and Gynecology. *Radiol. Clin. North Am.* 20:311–323, 1982.

Fiske C.E., Filly R.A.: Ultrasound evaluation of the normal and abnormal fetal neural axis, in Callen P.W. (ed.): *Ultrasonography in Obstetrics and Gynecology*. Philadelphia, W.B. Saunders Co., 1983, pp. 97–112.

# CHAPTER 6

# Thorax

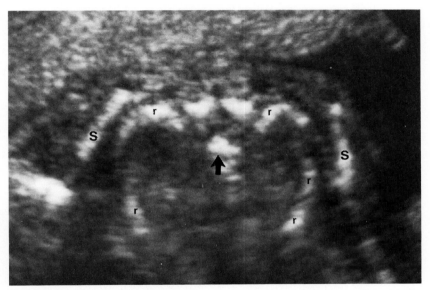

**Fig 6–1.**—Bony thorax; scapula, ribs. Transverse section through the mid-upper thorax delineates the three ossification centers within one vertebral segment *(arrow)* and portions of several ribs *(r)*. Note the position of the blade of the scapulae *(S)* external to the ribs, and surrounded by hypoechoic muscle.

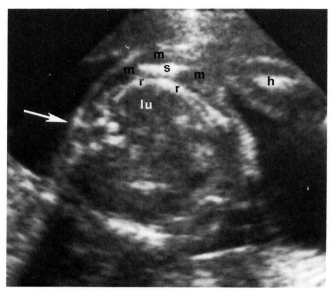

**Fig 6–2.**—Bony thorax; shoulder, 20 weeks. Oblique transverse section shows the scapula *(s)* surrounded by the thick hypoechoic musculature of the shoulder girdle *(m)*. The adjacent arm with a short segment of humerus *(h)* is noted. *r* = rib, *lu* = lung, *arrow* indicates spine.

**Fig 6–3.**—Bony thorax; shoulder, ribs. Oblique coronal section through the upper thorax reveals the y-shaped scapula *(s)* surrounded by the hypoechoic muscles of the shoulder girdle. The distal clavicle *(c)* is noted in addition to multiple ribs *(arrows)*. H = head.

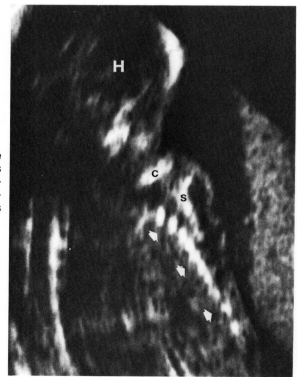

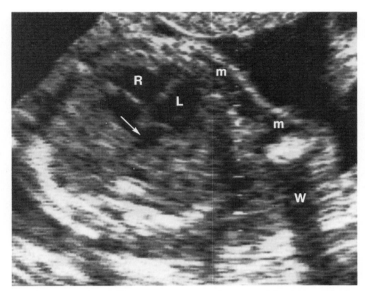

**Fig 6–4.**—Pectoralis muscles. Transverse section of the thorax viewed from below demonstrates a four-chamber view of the heart. *L* = left ventricle. *R* = right ventricle. *Arrow* indicates flow direction through the foramen ovale. The normal prominence of the hypoechoic pectoralis muscles extending from the anterior chest to the left shoulder girdle is appreciated *(m)*. *W* = shadow from proximal left humerus.

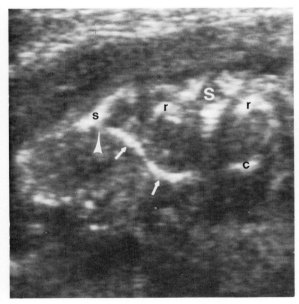

**Fig 6–5.**—Clavicle, acromioclavicular (AC) joint. Axial section, upper thorax. The anterior, curvilinear clavicle *(arrows)* is separated from the acromial process of the scapula *(s)* by the intervening AC joint *(arrowhead)*. Portions of the thoracic spine *(S)*, proximal ends of the first ribs *(r)*, and left clavicle *(c)* are seen.

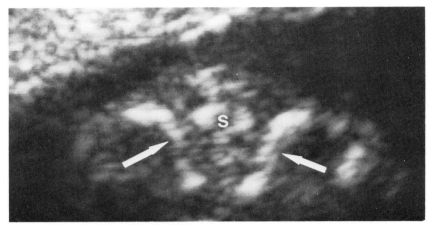

**Fig 6–6.**—Clavicles, 15 weeks. Transverse section at the thoracic inlet demonstrates the spine *(S)* and both clavicles *(arrows)* in close proximity.

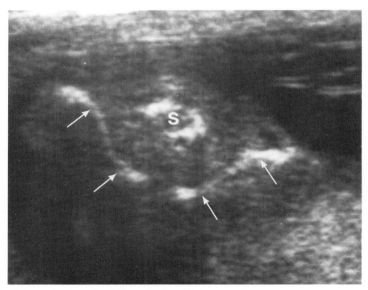

**Fig 6–7.**—Clavicles, 21 weeks. Transverse section through both the clavicles *(arrows)* and the spine *(S)* reveals interval elongation and more curvature in the clavicles compared to Figure 6–6. Due to the curved nature of the clav- icles, they are difficult to image either singularly or bilaterally in their entirety. The importance of their identification is in exclusion of some skeletal abnormalities with clavicular involvement.

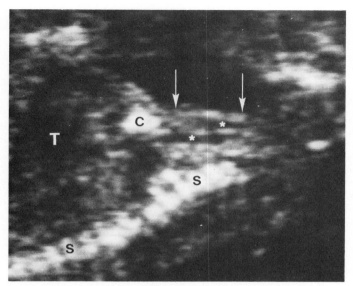

**Fig 6–8.**—Transverse clavicle, 19 weeks. Longitudinal scan through the upper thorax *(T)* and neck *(arrows)* delineates the anteriorly positioned clavicle *(C)* in cross-section, and a portion of the spine *(S)* posteriorly. Great vessels *(∗)* within the neck course just posterior to the clavicle.

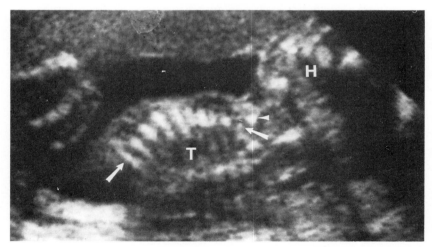

**Fig 6–9.**—Ribs. Longitudinal image through the fetal head *(H)* and thorax *(T)* reveals short segments of multiple ribs seen as echogenic linear structures *(between arrows).* Due to the curvilinear nature of ribs, it is impossible to image significant segments of multiple ribs simultaneously. *Arrowhead* indicates clavicle in cross-section.

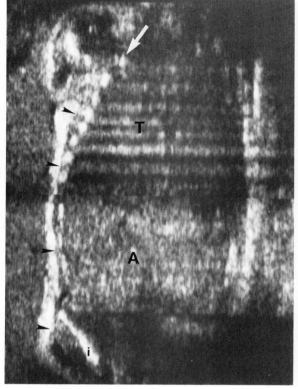

**Fig 6–10.**—Ribs, chest wall. Coronal image through the thorax *(T)* and abdomen *(A)* shows multiple ribs in cross-section *(arrow)*, casting shadows across the thorax. Hypoechoic chest wall musculature *(arrowheads)* surrounds the ribs and is contiguous with abdominal wall musculature that extends to blend with the muscles around the iliac crest *(i)*.

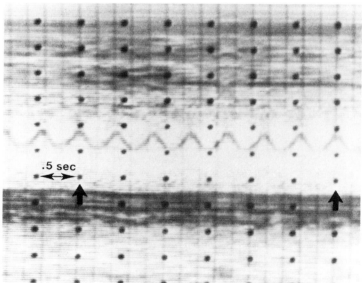

**Fig 6–11.**—M-mode tracing of fetal cardiac activity, 28 weeks. A regular sinus rhythm and a normal rate of 140 beats per minute are apparent. [One-half-second time interval exists between adjacent *vertical rows of dots.* Seven beats occur over the three-second interval indicated *between the wide arrows,* indicating a heart rate of 140 beats per minute.] Documentation of cardiac activity either by video or M-mode echocardiography may be important in some cases. If questions of AV block exist, separate rates should be obtained from the atria and the ventricles.

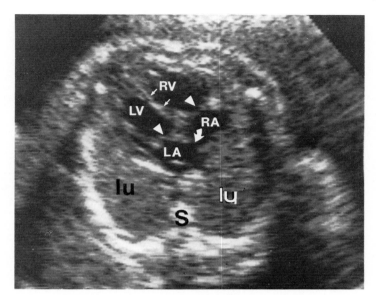

**Fig 6–12.**—Heart, four-chamber view. The four-chamber view of the heart is obtained in a transverse or angled transverse scan of the thorax. Overall, the heart occupies about one third of the cross-sectional area of the thorax in a transverse section. The internal anatomy is best appreciated when the fetal trunk points anteriorly without intervening bony structures in the scan plane. The right ventricle *(RV)* is the most anterior chamber while the left atrium *(LA)* is the most posterior and closest to the spine. *LV* = left ventricle, *RA* = right atrium. The interventricular septum *(small arrows)* separates the ventricles which are of approximately equal size. The foramen ovale *(curved arrow)* connects the atria, which are also of approximately equal size. The mitral and tricuspid valves *(arrowheads)* are closed. *lu* = lungs, *S* = spine.

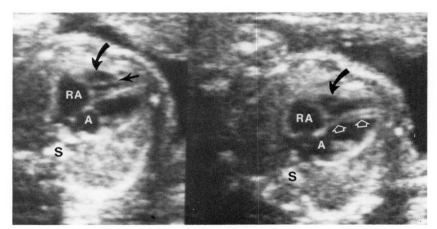

**Fig 6–13.**—Heart, papillary muscle, interventricular septum, 24 weeks. Two four-chamber views of the heart. The left atrium *(A)* is the most posterior chamber and the right ventricle *(curved arrows)*, the most anterior chamber. *RA* = right atrium. A papillary muscle is seen in the right ventricle *(straight arrow)*. The interventricular septum *(open arrows)* is intact. *S* = spine.

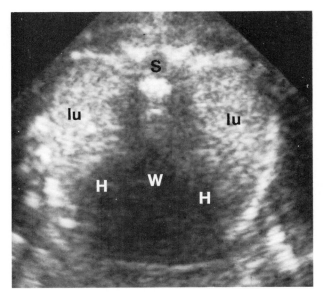

**Fig 6–14.**—Heart imaging, technical problems. Transverse section of the thorax at 26 weeks with the fetus in the prone position. It may be difficult or impossible to obtain significant structural information about the heart *(H)* when it is shadowed *(W)* by the ribs and spine *(S)*. Changing transducer position should still allow for determination of cardiac rate and rhythm, however. *lu* = lungs.

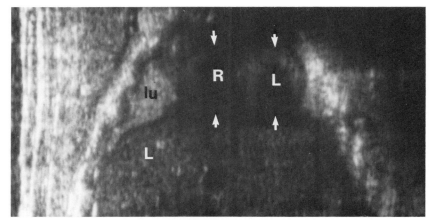

**Fig 6–15.**—Heart, short axis view. Both the right *(R)* and left *(upper L)* lateral ventricles are cut transversely, demonstrating equal chamber size and wall thickness *(arrows)*. Note the normal echogenic immature lung *(lu)* in contrast with the less echogenic liver *(lower L)*.

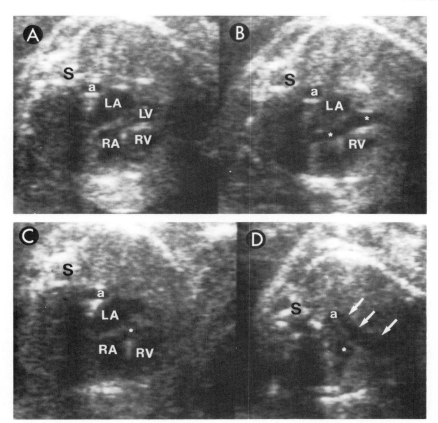

**Fig 6–16.**—Aortic and pulmonic outflow tracts, ductus arteriosus, 28 weeks. **A,** high four-chamber view. **B,** angling cephalad from **A;** the aortic outflow tract, aortic root, and proximal aortic arch (∗) are seen arising from the left ventricle and passing to the right between the left atrium and the right ventricle *(LA)*. **C,** transverse section just cephalad to **A** reveals a three-chamber view surrounding the aortic root (∗) which has already arisen from the left ventricle at a lower level. **D,** angling cephalad from **C** demonstrates the outflow tract arising from the right ventricle extending to the left and anterior to the aortic root (∗), as the left pulmonary artery and the ductus arteriosus *(arrows)* extend into the descending aorta *(a). LA =* left atrium, *RA =* right atrium, *LV =* left ventricle, *RV =* right ventricle, *a =* descending aorta, *S =* spine. It is important to note that the aortic outflow tract and the arch cross to the right of the midline, as opposed to the pulmonic outflow tract which courses anterior to the aorta and crosses to the left of midline.

**Fig 6–17.**—Ductus arteriosus. Transverse oblique section through the fetal thorax demonstrates the pulmonary outflow tract/left pulmonary artery (P), and the prominent ductus arteriosus (arrowheads) leading into the descending thoracic aorta (A). Note the normal orientation of the pulmonary outflow tract arising anterior to the ascending aorta (AA) and extending from right to left. W = shadow from the spine, R = right lateral thoracic wall, rib.

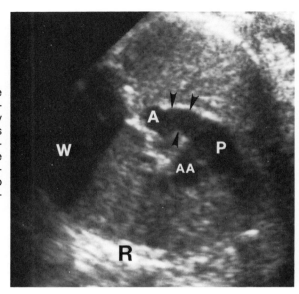

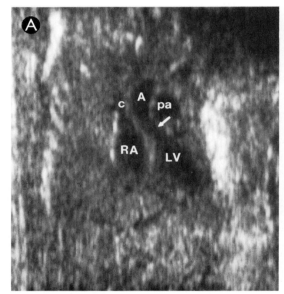

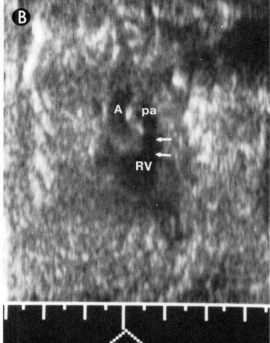

**Fig 6–18.**—Aortic and pulmonary outflow tracts. **A,** coronal image through the mid-heart shows the left ventricle (LV) contiguous with the aortic outflow tract (arrow) and ascending aortic arch (A) which are directed towards the right. RA = right atrium, c = superior vena cava, pa = pulmonary artery. **B,** coronal image anterior to **A** demonstrates the right ventricle (RV), with the right ventricular outflow tract (arrows) and main pulmonary artery (pa) extending to the left. A = ascending aortic arch. Identification of such normal vascular relationships is important in excluding transposition of the great vessels.

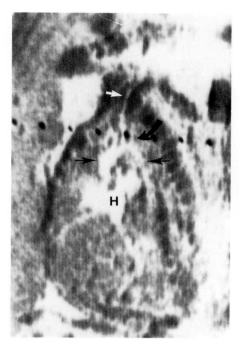

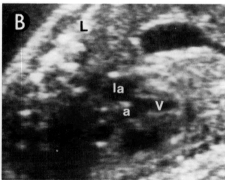

Fig 6–19.—Aortic arch and major branches. The entire arch of the aorta *(straight black arrows)* is imaged in an oblique longitudinal plane. The major branches to the upper body can be seen arising from the transverse arch *(curved arrow)*, with one vessel followed well into the neck *(white arrow). H* = heart.

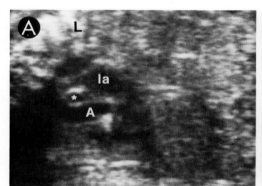

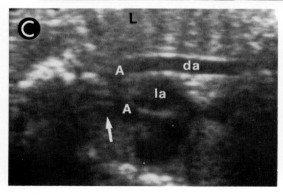

Fig 6–20.—Aortic outflow tract, root, arch, and descending aorta. Longitudinal oblique images through the fetal thorax. **A,** aortic root/ascending aortic arch *(A)* is seen to the right of and superior to the pulmonary artery *(\*). la* = left atrium. **B,** aortic outflow tract/root *(a),* which has a common wall with the left atrium *(la),* is seen coming off of the left ventricle *(V).* **C,** aortic arch *(A)* and descending aorta *(da)* are shown wrapping around the left atrium *(la).* The major vessels arising from the arch are indicated by an *arrow.*

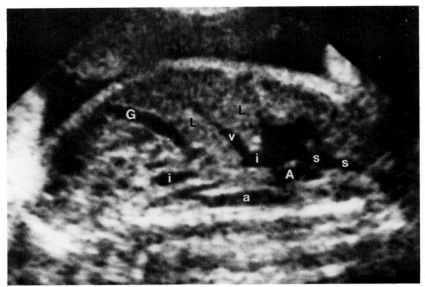

**Fig 6–21.**—Vena cava, 33 weeks. The inferior vena cava (IVC)*(i)* and superior vena cava *(s)* are seen entering the right atrium. A hepatic vein *(v)* courses obliquely through the liver into the sub-phrenic IVC. The gallbladder *(G)* is caudad to the liver *(L)*. In longitudinal section the gallbladder can be differentiated from the umbilical vein by its extrahepatic location, a more posterior proximal extension, and a lack of communication with the umbilical cord. *a* = aorta, *A* = left atrium.

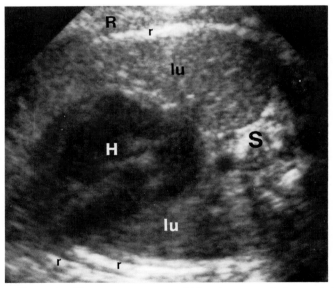

**Fig 6–22.**—Lungs, 33 weeks. Transverse section through thorax. The fetal heart *(H)* fills a large portion of the anterior and mid-thorax while mid-level echogenic lungs *(lu)* are noted postero-laterally. *R* = right, *S* = spine, *r* = ribs.

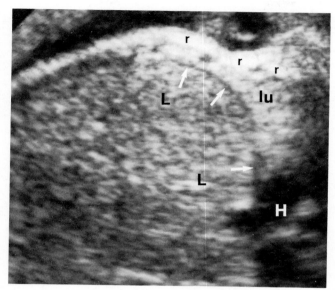

**Fig 6–23.**—Diaphragm and lungs, 28 weeks. Coronal section through the lower thorax and abdomen. The fetal diaphragm *(arrows)* is seen as a thin hypoechoic band between the lung *(lu)* and the liver *(L)*. The hypoechoic character of the diaphragm is similar to other fetal musculature. Note that the echogenicity of the lung is greater than that of the liver at this gestational age. *H* = heart, *r* = ribs.

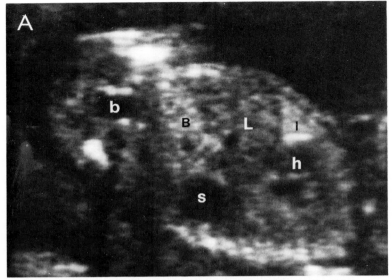

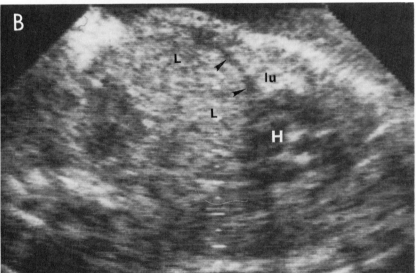

**Fig 6–24.**—Lung maturity. Coronal/longitudinal scans. **A,** fetal lung *(l)* is considerably more echogenic than liver *(L). h* = heart, *s* = stomach, *b* = bladder, *B* = bowel. **B,** fetal lung *(lu)* is slightly more echogenic than the right lobe of the liver *(L).* The hypoechoic diaphragm *(arrowheads)* separates these two organs. *H* = heart. *Continued.*

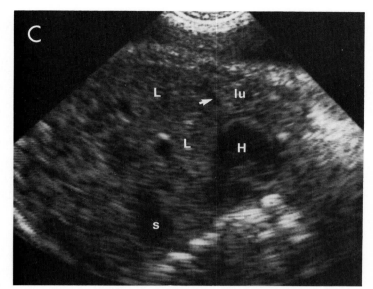

**Fig 6–24 *Cont.*—C,** if the hypoechoic diaphragm *(arrow)* were not present between the liver *(L)* and lung *(lu)*, they would appear as one organ as their echogenicity is equal. *H* = heart, *s* = stomach. Some preliminary work suggests that functional fetal lung maturity can be predicted sonographically by documenting a reduction in lung echogenicity from an immature pattern of echogenicity greater than liver to a mature pattern where lung and liver echotexture are comparable.

## REFERENCES

Allan L.D., Tynan M.J., Campbell S., et al.: Echocardiographic and anatomical correlates in the fetus. *Br. Heart J.* 44:444–451, 1980.

Axel L.: Real-time sonography of fetal cardiac anatomy. *A.J.R.* 141:283–288, 1983.

Elejalde B.R., de Elejalde M.M., Martinez D.P.: Ruling out tetralogy of Fallot at 21 weeks of gestation. *Rev. Brasil. Genet.* 6:347–351, 1983.

Filkins K.A., Brown T.F., Levine O.R.: Real time ultrasonic evaluation of the fetal heart. *Int. J. Gynaecol. Obstet.* 19:35–39, 1981.

Jeanty P., Romero R., Cantraine F., et al.: Fetal cardiac dimensions: a potential tool for the diagnosis of congenital heart defects. *J. Ultrasound Med.* 3:359–364, 1984.

Jeanty P., Romero R., Hobbins J.C.: Vascular anatomy of the fetus. *J. Ultrasound Med.* 3:113–122, 1984.

Jeffrey R.B., Laing F.C.: High-resolution real-time sonography of fetal cardiovascular anatomy. *J. Ultrasound Med.* 1:249–251, 1982.

Kleinman C.S., Donnerstein R.L., Jaffe C.C., et al.: Fetal echocardiography. *Am. J. Cardiol.* 51:237–243, 1983.

Knochel J.Q., Lee T.G., Melendez M.G., et al.: Fetal anomalies involving the thorax and abdomen, in Callen P.W. (ed.): *Ultrasonography in Obstetrics and Gynecology.* Philadelphia, W.B. Saunders Co., pp. 61–80, 1983.

Manning F.A., Heaman M., Boyce D., et al.: Intrauterine fetal tachypnea. *Obstet. Gynecol.* 58:398–400, 1981.

McCallum W.D.: Fetal cardiac anatomy and vascular dynamics. *Clin. Obstet. Gynecol.* 24:837–849, 1981.

Sahn D.J., Lange L.W., Allen H.D., et al.: Quantitative real-time cross-sectional echocardiography in the developing normal human fetus and newborn. *Circulation* 62:588–597, 1980.

Wheeler T., Murrills A.: Patterns of fetal heart rate during normal pregnancy. *Br. J. Obstet. Gynaecol.* 85:18–27, 1978.

# CHAPTER 7

# Abdomen and Pelvis

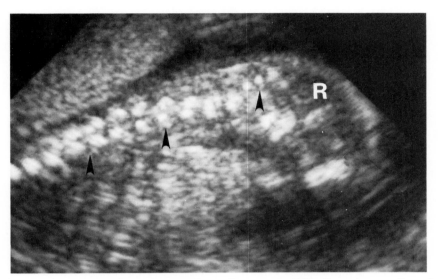

**Fig 7–1.**—Lumbosacral spine, 20 weeks. Prone sagittal section through the ossification centers of the lumbosacral spine *(arrowheads).* R = rump. With the spine positioned anteriorly, delineation of specific structures within the abdomen and pelvis is more difficult.

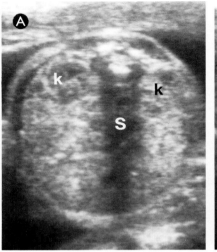

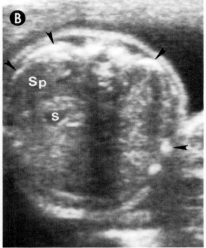

**Fig 7–2.**—Transverse prone upper abdomen, 27 weeks. **A,** fetal kidneys *(k)* are identified as bilateral hypoechoic paraspinal structures. The three ossification centers of the upper lumbar spine are seen with distal shadowing *(S).* **B,** transverse section at a higher level than **A** shows the midline lower thoracic spinal ossification centers with adjacent ribs *(arrowheads)* identified peripherally within the hypoechoic musculature of the abdominal wall. *Sp* = spleen. *S* = stomach.

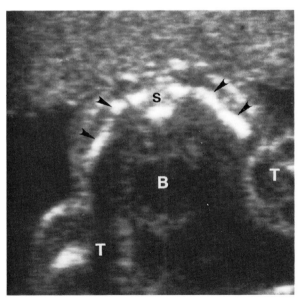

**Fig 7–3.**—Sacrum, iliac crests, SI joints. Axial section through pelvis delineating the three ossification centers of the sacrum *(S)* and the iliac crests *(arrowheads)* with the intervening SI joints. Proximal thighs *(T)* can be seen flexed on the abdomen. *B* = bladder.

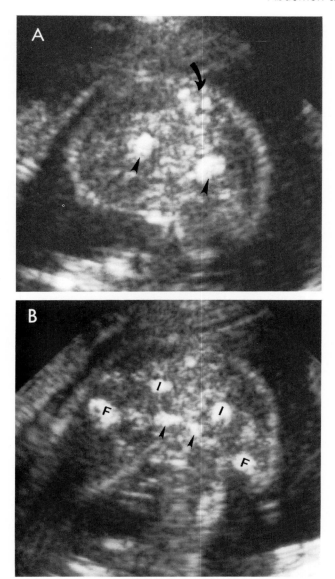

**Fig 7–4.**—Ischium, pubis, sacrum, 20 weeks. **A,** axial section through the low pelvis demonstrates three ossification centers within the sacral spine *(curved arrow)* and the ischial ossification centers *(arrowheads)* surrounded by hypoechoic pelvic musculature. **B,** lower axial section includes the proximal femurs *(F)* within the thighs. The central ischial ossification centers *(I)* are again seen as are the smaller, more anterior and medial ossification centers of the pubic bones *(arrowheads)*.

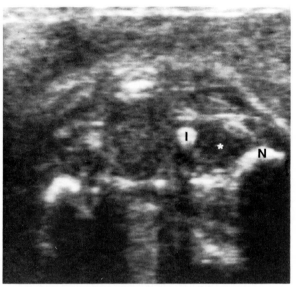

**Fig 7–5.**—Cartilaginous femoral head. Axial section through the ossified ischium *(I)* and proximally femoral neck *(N)* delineates the hypo-echoic cartilage of the developing femoral head *(∗)*.

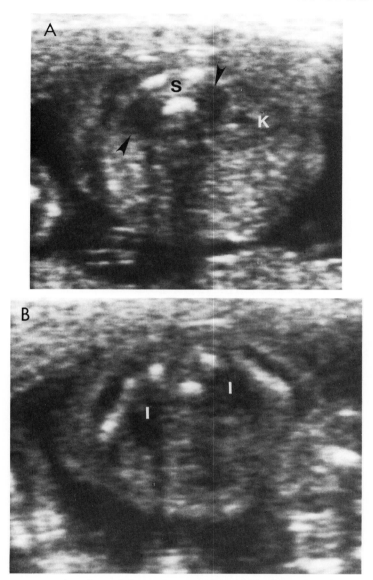

**Fig 7–6.**—Psoas muscle. **A,** axial section through the mid-abdomen and lumbar spine ossification centers *(S)*. Hypoechoic paraspinal structures represent the psoas muscles *(arrowheads)*. An adjacent kidney with minimal urine in the collecting system is noted *(K)*. **B,** lower axial section within the pelvis demonstrates the hypoechoic iliopsoas muscle *(I)* within the iliac fossa, adjacent to the spine. Symmetrical hypoechoic muscles should not be mistaken for masses arising from within the retroperitoneum or for dilated bowel.

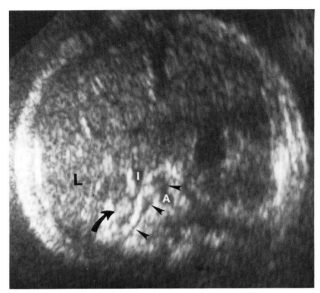

**Fig 7–7.**—Diaphragmatic crus, 34 weeks. Transverse section through the upper abdomen delineates the right crus of the diaphragm *(arrowheads)* as a hypoechoic structure, thin posteriorly with a prominent anterior bulge. The right adrenal gland *(arrow)* and the IVC *(I)* are seen between the crus and the liver *(L). A* = aorta.

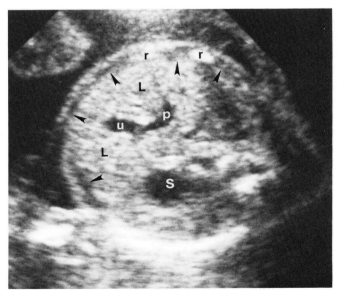

**Fig 7–8.**—Abdominal wall musculature, pseudoascites, 26 weeks. Transverse section through the liver *(L).* A hypoechoic band *(arrowheads)* between the liver and the echogenic skin has been termed "pseudoascites." In this case, this represents hypoechoic abdominal musculature, for in its posterior extension it can be seen to surround fetal ribs *(r). S* = stomach. *u* = umbilical vein. *p* = portal vein/portal sinus.

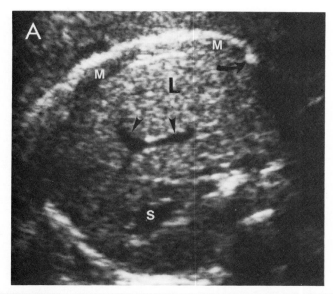

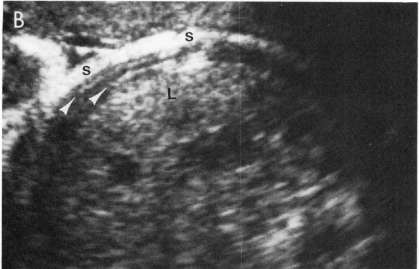

**Fig 7–9.**—Abdominal musculature, 34 weeks. **A,** transverse section through the liver *(L)* delineates umbilical vein entering the portal venous system *(arrowheads).* There is a prominent hypoechoic subcutaneous muscle layer *(M),* with a portion of one rib *(arrow)* noted posteriorly. This represents an exaggerated example of pseudoascites. *S* = stomach. **B,** close-up scan of the abdominal wall musculature between the liver *(L)* and subcutaneous tissue *(S)* reveals internal curvilinear echoes *(arrowheads)* representing fascial planes between the three layers of abdominal musculature (transversalis abdominis, internal oblique, and external oblique muscles).

**Fig 7–10.**—Abdominal musculature, subcutaneous tissue, 34 weeks. Transverse section of right side of abdomen shows the normal echogenic skin/subcutaneous tissues *(S)* measuring 3–4 mm in thickness. Abdominal wall musculature can be seen as a hypoechoic band *(arrowheads)* lateral to the liver *(L)* and kidney *(K)*.

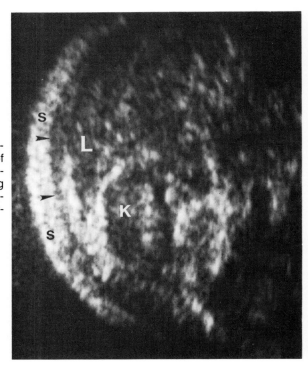

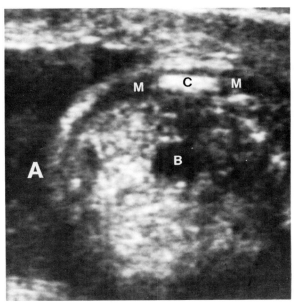

**Fig 7–11.**—Pelvic musculature. Transverse oblique section through the lower abdomen anteriorly and pelvis posteriorly reveals the echogenic iliac crest *(C)* lying within the thick hypoechoic musculature *(M)* of the lateral pelvis. The bladder *(B)* appears more posterior than usual due to the upwardly angled orientation of the scan. *A* = anterior.

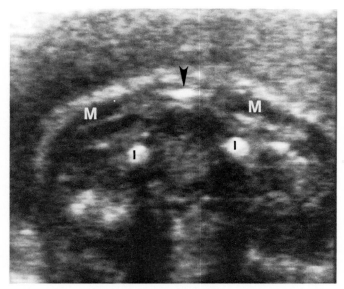

**Fig 7–12.**—Posterior pelvic musculature. Axial section below the iliac crests, through the gluteal musculature *(M),* which is separated by linear, echogenic fascial planes. A small sacral segment *(arrowhead)* and brightly echogenic and shadowing ischial ossification centers *(I)* are noted.

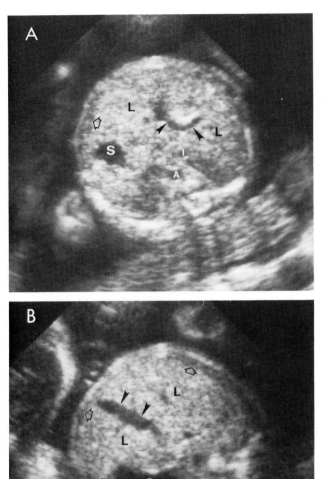

**Fig 7–13.**—Liver, stomach, umbilical vein, abdominal circumference, 23 weeks. **A,** appropriate section for abdominal circumference measurement. Circular axial section, symmetric with short rib segments at level of the junction of the umbilical vein with the portal vein/portal sinus *(arrowheads).* **B,** inappropriate section for abdominal circumference. Oblique and downwardly angled transverse section shows too long of a segment of umbilical vein *(arrowheads)* extending through the liver *(L)* towards the lower anterior abdominal wall (see Fig 7–14). The abdomen appears ovoid and a lcng segment of rib *(r)* is identified, indicating an oblique scan. The liver occupies a large percentage of the abdomen at this level, the left lobe being quite prominent in the fetus. The stomach *(S)* is seen posterior to the left lobe in the left upper quadrant. Hypoechoic abdominal musculature (pseudoascites) indicated with *arrows. A* = aorta. *I* = inferior vena cava.

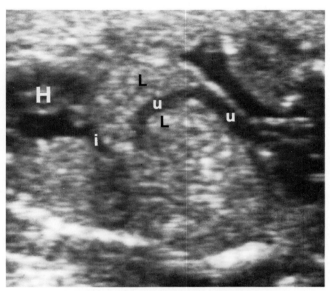

**Fig 7–14.**—Umbilical vein. Midline sagittal section through the abdomen and lower thorax demonstrates the umbilical vein *(u)* coursing from the cord insertion at the umbilicus through the anterior abdomen until it dives obliquely through the liver parenchyma *(L)* to reach the left portal vein. It is apparent that a true transverse section of the fetal abdomen obtained for an abdominal circumference measurement must be obtained at the point where only a short segment of umbilical vein is seen to enter the left portal vein. If a long segment of umbilical vein is imaged within the liver, the transverse section will be too ovoid and not truly axial. *H* = heart, *i* = inferior vena cava.

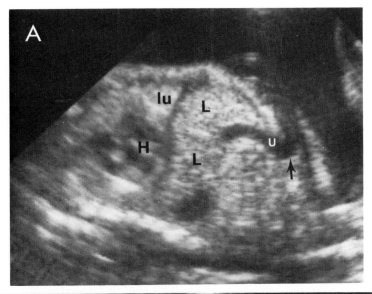

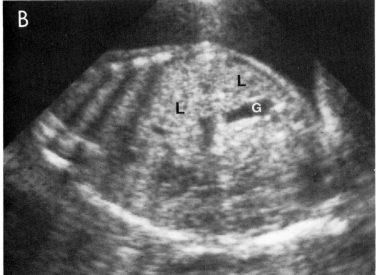

**Fig 7–15.**—Liver, gallbladder, umbilical vein, 23 weeks. Sequential right longitudinal images through the trunk. **A,** midline section shows the umbilical vein *(u)* coursing from its insertion at the umbilicus *(arrow)* anteriorly through the abdomen to enter the left lobe of the liver *(L)* and course posteriorly-superiorly. The hypoechoic diaphragm, contiguous anteriorly with anterior trunk musculature, is seen separating the liver from lung *(lu)* and heart *(H).* No ribs are seen anteriorly in the thorax, allowing for optimal visualization of intrathoracic structures. **B,** to the right, the gallbladder *(G),* typically somewhat teardrop-shaped, lies posteroinferiorly to the liver *(L).* It extends from the region of the porta hepatis and may contact the anterior abdominal wall. *Continued.*

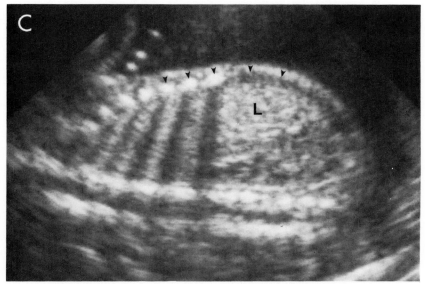

**Fig 7–15 Cont.—C,** further to the right, multiple ribs with distal shadowing can be appreciated. The musculature in which the ribs lie is contiguous with the hypoechoic musculature *(arrowheads)* of the anterior abdominal wall which may simulate ascites (pseudoascites) on transverse sections. *L* = right lobe of liver.

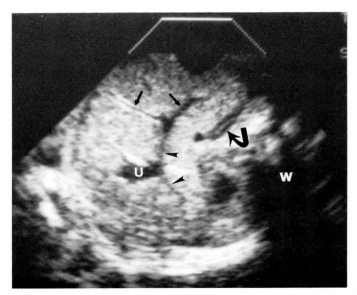

**Fig 7–16.**—Hepatic portal venous anatomy, adrenal gland. Transverse section through the fetal liver. The umbilical vein *(U)* traverses the left lobe of the liver anteriorly to join the left portal vein at the junction of its medial and lateral segments *(arrowheads).* The left portal vein can be traced to the right where the right main portal vein and its anterior and posterior divisions *(small arrows)* are noted. The right adrenal gland, a thin hypoechoic structure with a central liner echo *(curved arrow),* is seen posterior to and in contact with the inferior vena cava. *W* = shadowing from spine.

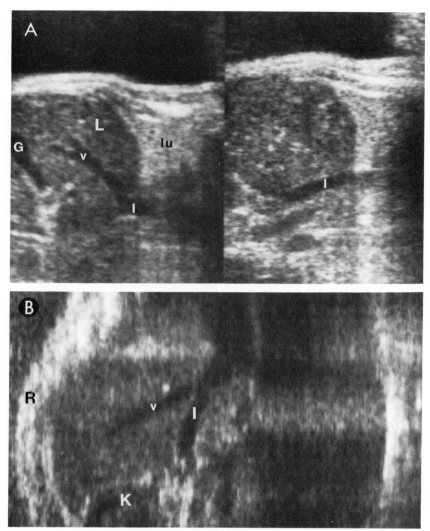

**Fig 7–17.**—Hepatic veins, gallbladder, inferior vena cava (IVC). **A, left,** longitudinal oblique image through the upper abdomen and lower thorax in the plane of the interlobar fissure of the liver. The middle hepatic vein *(v)* traverses that fissure within the liver *(L)* to enter the inferior vena cava *(I)* just caudal to the level of the diaphragm. The fetal gallbladder *(G),* which arises from the inferior aspect of the interlobar fissure, can be seen at the caudal margin of the liver. Lung echogenicity *(lu)* is greater than that of liver. **Right,** angling further to the right shows a long segment of IVC *(I)* traversing the liver. **B,** coronal section through the liver shows the right hepatic vein *(v)* coursing obliquely through the liver to enter the inferior vena cava *(I).* K = upper pole of right kidney. R = right abdominal wall.

Fig 7–18.—Gallbladder, umbilical vein, 32 weeks. Angled transverse scan of the upper abdomen. A long segment of umbilical vein *(U)* can be seen extending from the anterior abdominal wall into the liver. The umbilical vein lies essentially directly opposite from the spine and penetrates into the liver to join the left portal vein. Its caliber is relatively uniform throughout its intra-abdominal course. This is contrasted with the gallbladder *(G)* which lies to the right of midline, frequently does not reach the anterior abdominal wall, does not significantly penetrate the liver substance, and usually has a teardrop shape. The differentiation of these structures is important when obtaining an abdominal circumference measurement based on specific *umbilical vein/portal vein* anatomy. There is no significance to failure to identify the gallbladder. Electronic calipers indicate an abdominal circumference was taken on this section; however, a long segment of umbilical vein usually indicates an angled, and hence inappropriate, section for determining abdominal circumference. *W* = shadowing from spine.

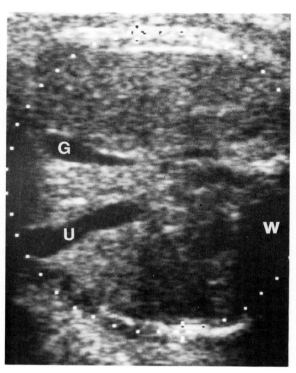

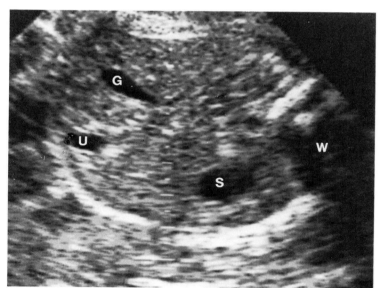

Fig 7–19.—Stomach, gallbladder. Transverse section through the upper abdomen reveals the only normally seen, major fluid-filled structures. *S* = stomach. *G* = gallbladder. *U* = umbilical vein. The stomach should be identifiable in all fetuses from the second trimester, although it may be quite small. It ranges in shape from round to ovoid to slightly bean-shaped and may be imaged posteriorly to quite far anteriorly within the left upper quadrant (see Figs 7–13, 7–20, 7–38). Note that the umbilical vein lies directly opposite the spine (*W* = shadowing from spine), whereas the gallbladder lies to the right of midline. This section is too low for an abdominal circumference determination as the umbilical vein is still located anteriorly within the falciform ligament.

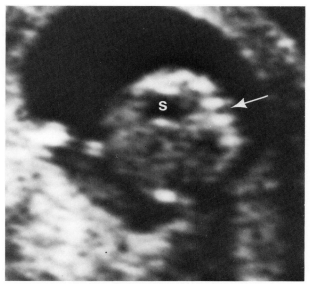

**Fig 7–20.**—Stomach, 14.5 weeks. Early identification of a 7-mm fluid-filled stomach *(S)* in the left upper quadrant, on transverse section. *Arrow* indicates spine. Specific non-fluid-filled structures are hard to identify early in pregnancy due to size and subject contrast constraints.

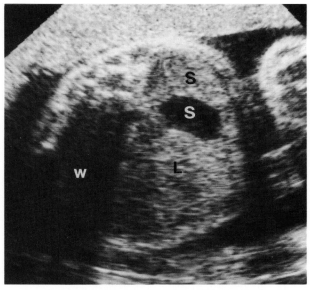

**Fig 7–21.**—Spleen, stomach. Transverse section at the level of the stomach *(white S)* shows a retrogastric solid structure representing the spleen *(black S)*. *W* = shadowing from the fetal spine. *L* = left lobe of liver.

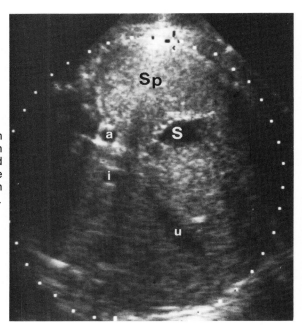

**Fig 7–22.**—Spleen. Transverse section through the upper abdomen reveals the spleen *(Sp)* as a posterior left upper quadrant solid structure of mid-level echoes separated from the stomach *(S)* by echogenic fat. The umbilical vein *(u)*, aorta *(a)*, and inferior vena cava *(i)* are seen.

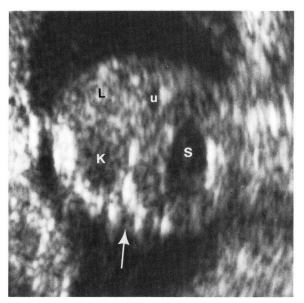

**Fig 7–23.**—Kidney, 15 weeks. Transverse section through the abdomen suggests a sonolucent right paraspinal structure (*K* = kidney) posterior to the liver *(L)*. Fetal kidneys are difficult to identify in the early second trimester, but may be suggested by the presence of round or ovoid sonolucent structures in a paraspinal location. By 20 weeks, at least one kidney is identifiable in most fetuses. *Arrow* indicates spine. *S* = stomach. *u* = umbilical vein.

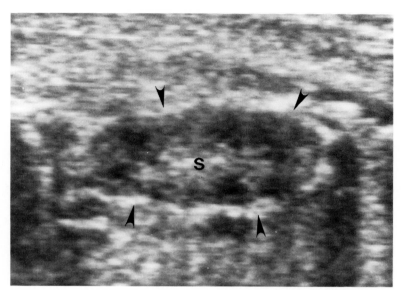

**Fig 7–24.**—Kidney, renal capsule, 33 weeks. Longitudinal section. By the early third trimester, renal margins are well delineated by the echogenic renal capsule *(arrowheads)*. The central renal sinus *(S)* is more echogenic than the surrounding renal parenchyma.

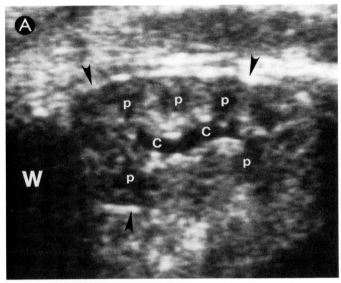

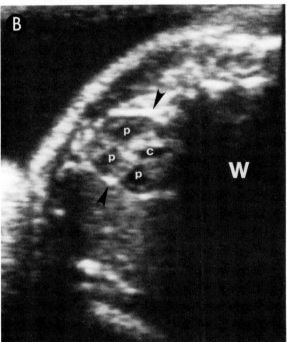

**Fig 7–25.**—Kidney, pyramids, collecting system, 31 weeks. Longitudinal **(A)** and transverse prone **(B)** scans. The kidney is outlined by an echogenic renal capsule *(arrowheads)*. Centrally within the kidney, the echogenic sinus is minimally separated by a normal amount of urine within the collecting system *(C)*. The hypoechoic pyramids *(p)* can be seen periodically located within the parenchyma, adjacent to the echogenic sinus. The remaining parenchymal echoes are mid-level between sinus and pyramids. *W* = shadowing from iliac crest **(A)** and spine **(B)**.

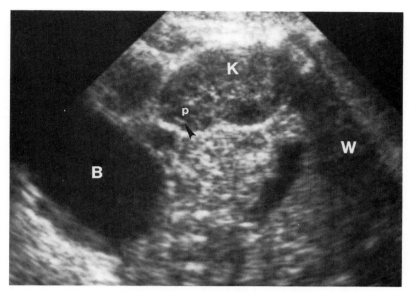

**Fig 7–26.**—Arcuate artery, bladder. Coronal image demonstrates the normal proximity of the urine-filled bladder *(B)* to the kidney *(K)*. An arcuate artery *(arrowhead)* is seen as an echogenic line between a pyramid *(p)* and adjacent cortex. There is some shadowing *(W)* of the upper pole from a superimposed rib.

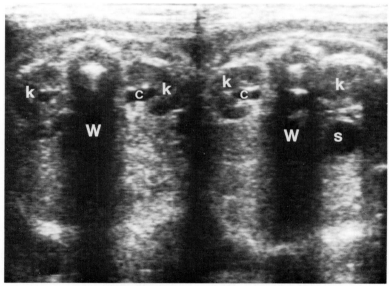

**Fig 7–27.**—Kidneys, renal pelvis, 35 weeks. Transverse prone sections through the fetal kidneys *(k)*. Right scan is at a higher level imaging the upper pole of the left kidney posterior to the stomach *(s)*. W = shadowing from spine. The renal pelvis *(c)* may appear very prominent in the third trimester and still be within normal limits. The more intrarenal portions of the collecting systems are generally not as prominent as the renal pelvis. Scanning over time will delineate the dynamic nature of urine flow through the kidney as changes in the degree of pelvic distention are documented.

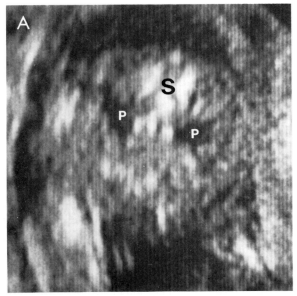

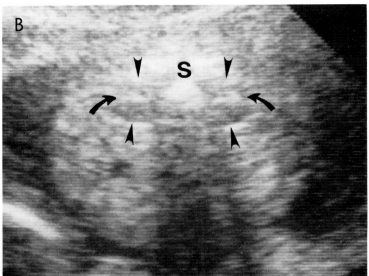

**Fig 7–28.**—Renal function. Transverse sections. **A,** initial scan demonstrates prominent dilatation of the renal pelvis *(P)* bilaterally. *S* = spine. **B,** repeat scan of the kidneys *(arrowheads)* five minutes later reveals interval resolution of the prominent renal pelvis, with no urine identifiable within the collecting systems and the sinus again appearing as compact echogenic areas *(curved arrows).* Concurrent imaging of the pelvis revealed increasing bladder size as the renal pelvis emptied. *S* = spine. This case indicates the importance of recognizing the normal prominent renal pelvis which can be delineated from the pathologically dilated pelvis by scanning over time.

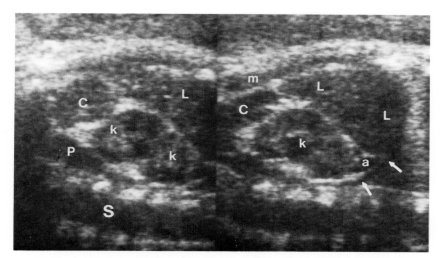

**Fig 7–29.**—Right renal relationships, adrenal gland, psoas muscle, 35 weeks. Coronal low **(left)** and high **(right)** scans through the right side of the abdomen demonstrate the kidney *(k)* surrounded by echogenic perirenal fat, liver *(L)*, right adrenal *(a),* and a portion of the ascending colon *(C)*. The right crus of the diaphragm *(arrows)* is a thin hypoechoic structure extending from the diaphragm down to wrap around the spine medial to the adrenal and upper pole of the kidney. The abdominal wall muscles *(m)* and psoas muscle *(P)* adjacent to the spine *(S)* are also hypoechoic structures that widen as they extend caudally.

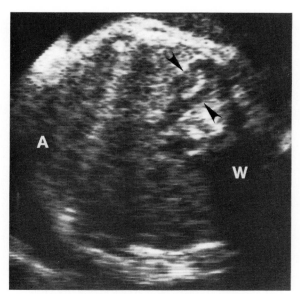

**Fig 7–30.**—Adrenal gland. Transverse upper abdominal section. The right adrenal gland is seen as a lenticular hypoechoic paraspinal structure with a linear echogenic core *(arrowheads).* This gland is rather plump and should not be mistaken for a fetal kidney. (Contrast with Fig 7–16.) *W* = shadowing from spine. *A* = anterior.

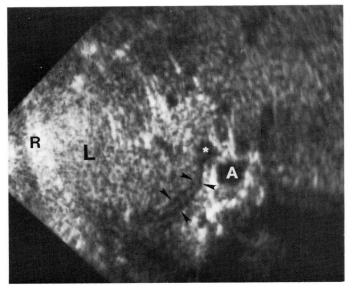

**Fig 7–31.**—Adrenal gland, term gestation. Transverse section through the upper abdomen shows a thin, curvilinear right adrenal gland *(arrowheads)* immediately posterior to the inferior vena cava *(\*)*. The outer portion of the adrenal is hypoechoic and the inner core is echogenic. *A* = aorta. *L* = liver. *R* = right lateral abdominal wall.

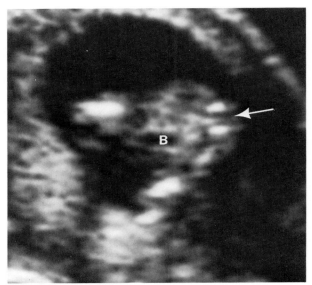

**Fig 7–32.**—Bladder, 14.5 weeks. Transverse image demonstrates a 4-mm fluid-filled bladder *(B)* anteriorly and low within the pelvis. *Arrow* indicates spine. Thighs/femurs are noted anteriorly. The natural contrast inherent in fluid-filled structures in the abdomen allows for visualizing the bladder at a very early stage. This may become important in the evaluation of various genitourinary (GU) tract abnormalities.

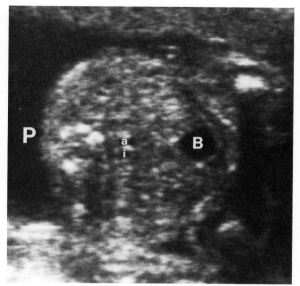

**Fig 7–33.**—Bladder. Angled axial image through the fetal pelvis at 22 weeks. In transverse section, the fetal bladder *(B)* is identified as a spherical or ovoid fluid-filled structure, low, midline, and anterior within the pelvis *(P)*. The aorta *(a)* and inferior vena cava *(i)* are seen anterior to the spine. The thighs/femurs are noted in flexed position anterior to the pelvis.

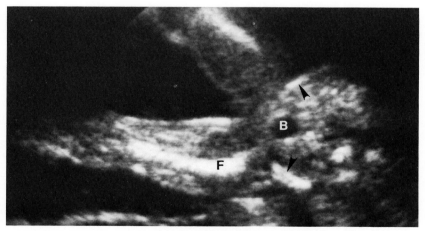

**Fig 7–34.**—Bladder, 18 weeks. Longitudinal section through the pelvis and thighs delineates the bladder *(B)* as a low-lying, midline, fluid-filled structure within the pelvis, located between the iliac crests *(arrowheads)*. The fluid-filled structure identified as bladder must be located within the expected margins of the fetal pelvis so as not to mistake a pocket of fluid tucked between the thighs as bladder. Pelvic bony landmarks are helpful in this determination. *F* = femur.

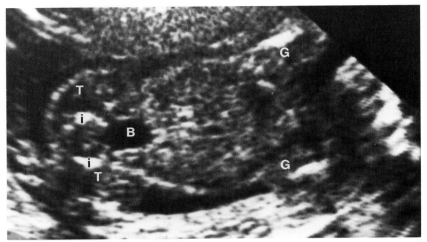

**Fig 7–35.**—Bladder. Coronal image of the fetal trunk demonstrates the fetal bladder *(B)* located low in the pelvis adjacent to the ischial ossification centers *(i)*. Proximal thighs *(T)* are noted. G = soft tissue and bones of the shoulder girdles.

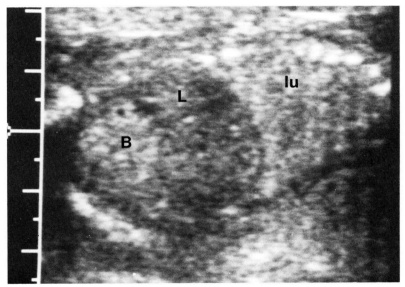

**Fig 7–36.**—Bowel, 16 weeks. Longitudinal section through the trunk. The liver *(L)* is less echogenic than the bowel *(B)* and lung *(lu)*. Through the second trimester, bowel frequently cannot be differentiated from liver based on echo texture alone. Occasionally, it is more echogenic than the adjacent liver, however, as in this case. It usually does not contain obvious amounts of fluid/meconium until the third trimester.

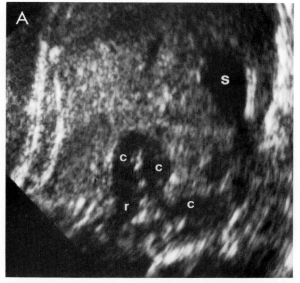

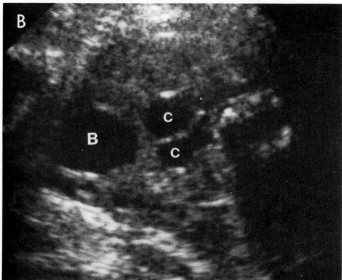

**Fig 7–37.**—Rectosigmoid colon, 30 weeks. **A,** coronal section through the abdomen and pelvis delineates a curved, tubular, sonolucent structure in the lower abdomen and pelvis, representing the sigmoid colon *(c)* and rectum *(r)*. The stomach *(S)* is seen in the left upper quadrant. **B,** transverse scan through the pelvis demonstrates two loops of sigmoid colon *(c)* posterior to the bladder *(B)*. Fetal colon is normally seen in the third trimester as hypoechoic tubular structures with internal low-level echoes. Occasionally haustrations can be identified. If the colon appears anechoic, dilated, or persistent in its distribution, the possibility of obstruction should be considered.

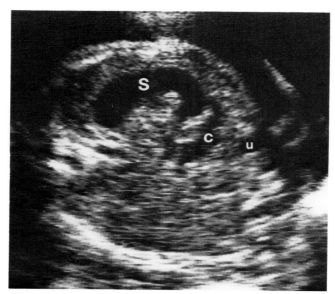

**Fig 7–38.**—Transverse colon, 28 weeks. Transverse oblique abdominal section. Anterior to the stomach *(S)* is a short segment of the fluid-filled transverse colon *(c)*. Haustrations are suggested by the irregular margins. The umbilical vein *(u)* can be seen anteriorly. Early in the third trimester, fluid-filled loops of colon are first becoming apparent.

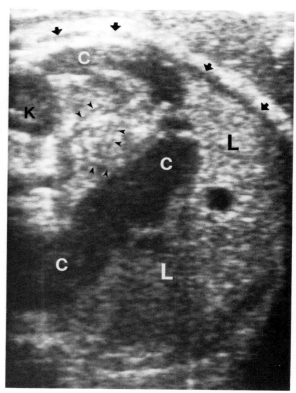

**Fig 7–39.**—Transverse colon, small bowel, 36 weeks. Transverse section through the upper abdomen. A large, hypoechoic, curved tubular structure of varied caliber represents the transverse colon *(C)* posterior to the liver *(L)*. Low level internal echoes represent meconium. Two linear echogenic bands traversing the lumen suggest haustrations. Between the colon and the left kidney *(K)* are multiple non-fluid-filled loops of small bowel. Several hypoechoic linear areas represent individual bowel walls *(arrowheads)*. *Arrows* indicate pseudoascites which can be seen to represent an anterior extension of the musculature which surrounds a rib more posteriorly.

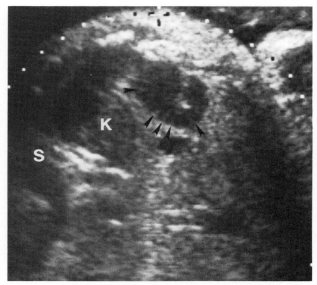

**Fig 7–40.**—Small bowel, 36 weeks. Transverse section through the upper abdomen shows a hypoechoic, curved, tubular structure representing fluid-filled small bowel. The valvulae conniventes can be appreciated *(arrowheads)*. Visualization of fluid-filled small bowel is unusual but, without undue dilatation or hyperactive peristalsis, is probably a normal variant. This would be supported by a stomach of normal size. *S* = spine. *K* = left kidney.

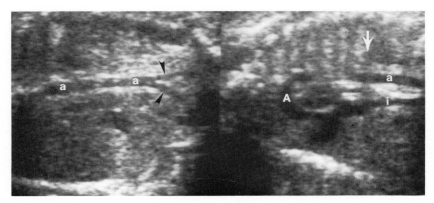

**Fig 7–41.**—Aorta, inferior vena cava (IVC), 28 weeks. Coronal images through abdomen and thorax. **Left,** abdominal aorta *(a)* seen to bifurcation into common iliac arteries *(arrowheads).* **Right,** *arrow* indicates approximate level of diaphragm. The upper abdominal portions of the aorta *(a)* and IVC *(i)* are seen. *A* = aortic arch.

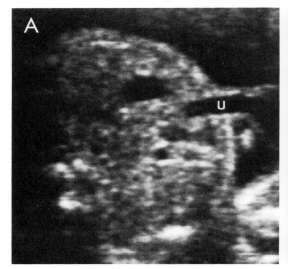

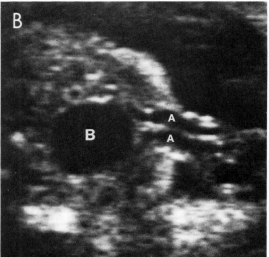

**Fig 7–42.**—Umbilical arteries and vein, umbilical cord, 24 weeks. Angled transverse sections through the fetal abdomen at the level of the cord insertion. **A,** the umbilical vein *(U)* is seen passing from the umbilical cord into the abdomen. **B,** both umbilical arteries *(A)* are identified in the cord before passing into the pelvis to branch laterally around the bladder *(B).*

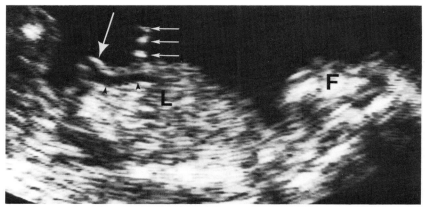

**Fig 7–43.**—Umbilical vein, umbilical cord, 17 weeks. Sagittal image. The umbilical vein within the cord enters the abdomen at the umbilicus *(large arrow),* and courses anteriorly through the abdomen *(arrowheads)* to enter the liver *(L).* The typical three parallel echo appearance of the umbilical cord within the amniotic cavity is appreciated *(small arrows). F* = face.

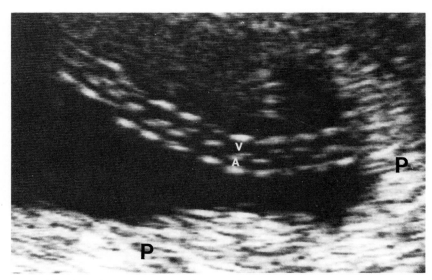

**Fig 7–44.**—Umbilical cord, 15.5 weeks. A longitudinal section through the umbilical cord demonstrates a marginal site of attachment to placenta (P). Multiple, periodic, "stacked" linear echoes represent vascular margins of the spiraling vessels within the cord. The larger space represents the vein (V), the smaller space an adjacent artery (A).

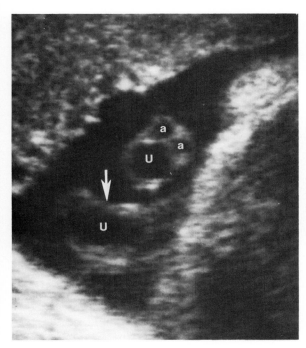

**Fig 7–45.**—Umbilical cord, 36 weeks. Transverse and oblique (arrow) sections through the umbilical cord demonstrate the larger umbilical vein (U) and the smaller umbilical arteries (a). More soft tissue (Wharton's jelly) surrounding the vessels is apparent than earlier in pregnancy. A transverse image is the most sensitive means for delineating the presence of three cord vessels, as longitudinal sections may prove confusing due to the spiral nature of the vessels.

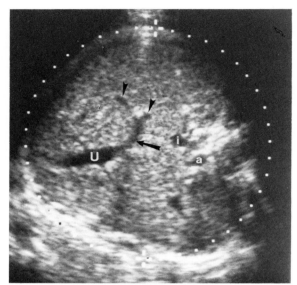

**Fig 7–46.**—Abdominal circumference, umbilical vein, portal sinus, 33 weeks. Transverse section through the liver shows the umbilical vein *(U)* joining the portal sinus (left portal vein, *arrow).* The anterior and posterior divisions of the right portal vein are apparent *(arrowheads).* Small tributary veins leading into the umbilical vein can be seen. *a* = aorta. *i* = IVC. This is an appropriate transverse section for determination of the abdominal circumference, i.e., at the level where the umbilical vein enters the left portal venous system. Abdominal circumference is used in consort with other fetal measurement parameters in the prediction of weight and evaluation for growth retardation. Obtaining a complete cross-section of the abdomen may be difficult, particularly in advanced pregnancies where a sector scanner is used and the fetus is positioned close to the anterior maternal abdominal wall. Electronic calipers can provide an approximation of the margins of the abdominal wall as in this case. An abdominal diameter can also be measured at this scanning level as indicated by the electronic calipers (+) on the right and left lateral aspects of the abdomen.

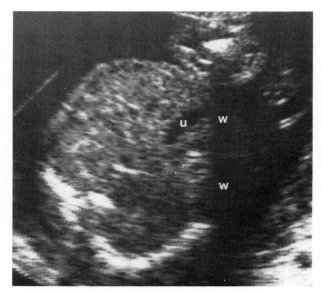

**Fig 7–47.**—Pitfall in abdominal circumference determination, 25 weeks. Transverse section through the upper abdomen at the level of the umbilical vein *(u)*. Shadowing *(w)* from an adjacent long bone has obscured a portion of the abdomen which could lead to an abnormally low measurement for the abdominal circumference if not recognized.

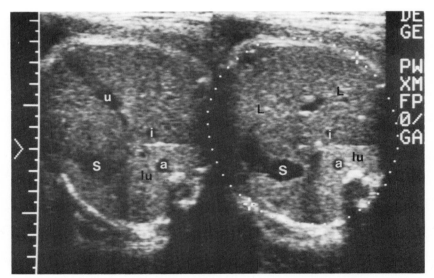

**Fig 7–48.**—Pitfall, abdominal circumference measurement, 33 weeks. Angled transverse sections of the fetal abdomen imaged from a lower point on the anterior abdominal wall to a higher level on the posterior thoracic wall are, as such, inappropriate for determination of abdominal circumference as indicated by electronic calipers on the right ( + ). One can discern this angling by the ovoid shape of the abdomen and significant components of the echogenic lung *(lu)* identified posteriorly about the spine. *L* = liver. *u* = umbilical vein. *S* = stomach. *a* = aorta. *i* = inferior vena cava.

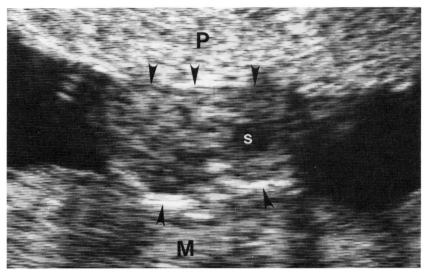

**Fig 7–49.**—Pitfall, abdominal measurements. Transverse section at 16 weeks demonstrates marked compression of the fetal abdomen (arrowheads) between the placenta (P) and posterior myometrium (M). The altered configuration of the abdomen would make determination of an abdominal diameter or circumference suboptimal. S = stomach.

## REFERENCES

Bertagnoli L., Lalatta F., Gallicchio R., et al.: Quantitative characterization of the growth of the fetal kidney. *J. C. U.* 11:349–356, 1983.

Bowie J.D., Rosenberg E.R., Andreotti R.F., et al.: The changing sonographic appearance of fetal kidneys during pregnancy. *J. Ultrasound Med.* 2:505–507, 1983.

Chinn D.H., Filly R.A., Callen P.W.: Ultrasonic evaluation of fetal umbilical and hepatic vascular anatomy. *Radiology* 144:153–157, 1982.

Cyr D.R.: Ultrasonic visualization of the fetal pancreas and hepatic venous circulation. *Med. Ultrasound* 7:27–31, 1983.

Deter R.L., Harrist R.B., Hadlock F.P., et al.: Fetal head and abdominal circumferences: I. Evaluation of measurement errors. *J. C. U.* 10:357–363, 1982.

Dubbins P.A., Kurtz A.B., Wapner R.J., et al.: Renal agenesis: spectrum of in utero findings. *J. C. U.* 9:189–193, 1981.

Eliezer S., Ester F., Ehud W., et al.: Fetal splenomegaly, ultrasound diagnosis of cytomegalovirus infection: a case report. *J. C. U.* 12:520–521, 1984.

Grannum P., Bracken M., Silverman R., et al.: Assessment of fetal kidney size in normal gestation by comparison of ratio of kidney circumference to abdominal circumference. *Am. J. Obstet. Gynecol.* 136:249–254, 1980.

Gross B.H., Filly R.A., Harter L.P.: Inability of relative fetal hepatic lobar size to diagnose intrauterine growth retardation. *J. Ultrasound Med.* 1:299–300, 1982.

Hadlock F.P., Deter R.L., Harrist R.B., et al.: Fetal abdominal circumference as a predictor of menstrual age. *A.J.R.* 139:367–370, 1982.

Jeanty P., Dramaix-Wilmet M., Elkhazen N., et al.: Measurement of fetal kidney growth on ultrasound. *Radiology* 144:159–162, 1982.

Jeanty P., Romero R., Hobbins J.C.: Vascular anatomy of the fetus. *J. Ultrasound Med.* 3:113–122, 1984.

Knochel J.O., Lee T.G., Melendez M.G., et al.: Fetal anomalies involving the thorax and abdomen, Symposium on Ultrasonography in Obstetrics and Gynecology. *Radiol. Clin. North Am.* 20:297–310, 1982.

Kurjak A., Kirkinen P., Latin V., et al.: Ultrasonic assessment of fetal kidney function in normal and complicated pregnancies. *Am. J. Obstet. Gynecol.* 141:266–270, 1981.

Lawson T.L., Foley W.D., Berland L.L., et al.: Ultrasonic evaluation of fetal kidneys. *Radiology* 138:153–156, 1981.

Lee T.G., Warren B.H.: Antenatal ultrasonic demonstration of fetal bowel. *Radiology* 124:471–474, 1977.

Morin F.R., Winsberg F.: The ultrasonic appearance of the umbilical cord. *J. C. U.* 6:324–326, 1978.

Morin F.R., Winsberg F.: Ultrasonic and radiographic study of the vessels of the fetal liver. *J. C. U.* 6:409–411, 1978.

Rosenthal S.J., Filly R.A., Callen P.W., et al.: Fetal pseudoascites. *Radiology* 131:195–197, 1979.

Rossavik I.K., Deter R.L.: The effect of abdominal profile shape changes on the estimation of fetal weight. *J. C. U.* 12:57–59, 1984.

Sarti D.A., Crandall B.F., Winter J., et al.: Correlation of biparietal and fetal body diameters: 12–26 weeks gestation. *A.J.R.* 137:87–91, 1981.

Skovbo P., Smith-Jensen S.: Hyperdistended fluid-filled bowel loops mimicking gastrointestinal atresia. *J. C. U* 9:463–465, 1981.

Tamura R.K., Sabbagha R.E.: Percentile ranks of sonar fetal abdominal circumference measurements. *Am. J. Obstet. Gynecol.* 138:475–479, 1980.

Woo J.S.K., Liang S.T., Wan C.W., et al.: Abdominal circumference vs abdominal area—which is better? *J. Ultrasound Med.* 3:101–105, 1984.

# CHAPTER 8

# Genitalia

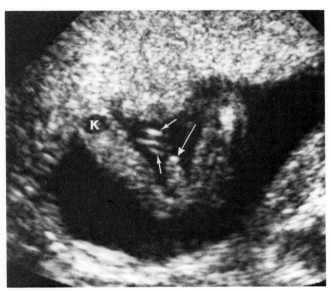

**Fig 8–1.**—Male, 16 weeks. A transverse section through the low pelvis, with thighs flexed, demonstrates the penis *(long arrow)* to be a solid structure as opposed to the adjacent cord *(short arrows)* which demonstrates the early, typical, three parallel echogenic line structure representing the margins of any two cord vessels. *K* = hypoechoic cartilage of knee joint. The determination of fetal gender is quite accurate from 20 weeks to term, if there is satisfactory visualization of the fetal peritoneum. Fetal factors such as presentation, lie, number, and activity, as well as placental position, fluid volume, and maternal size, all affect one's technical ability to adequately scan the fetal perineal region. When specific fetal genital structures are identified prior to 20 weeks, a diagnosis of sex can again be made; however, a large number of indeterminate examinations should be expected in this gestational age range. Male and female genitalia are not embryologically different until approximately 12 weeks gestational age, and even up to 20 weeks, there is considerable similarity between the scrotum and the labia majora. The most certain diagnosis will be made with the identification of the penis as in this case. The best scanning plans for determination of fetal gender are transverse or axial sections with mild degrees of sloping or angulation as necessary to appropriately image the peritoneal region. A potential pitfall in the diagnosis of fetal sex is the misinterpretation of the umbilical cord as a penis in a female fetus. The penis should appear as a solid structure, while the umbilical cord has internal fluid-filled areas corresponding to the normal three vessels.

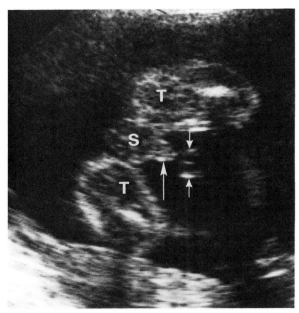

**Fig 8–2.**—Male, 26 weeks. Transverse section through the male genitalia demonstrates the scrotum *(S)* and portion of the penis *(long arrow)* projected between the proximal thighs *(T)*. Note the proximity of umbilical cord *(short arrows)*.

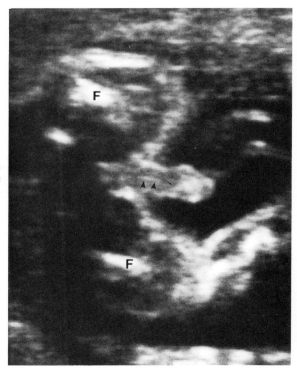

**Fig 8–3.**—Male urethra, 24 weeks. The penis is extended between the thighs. An echogenic central line probably represents the urethra *(arrowheads)*. F = femurs.

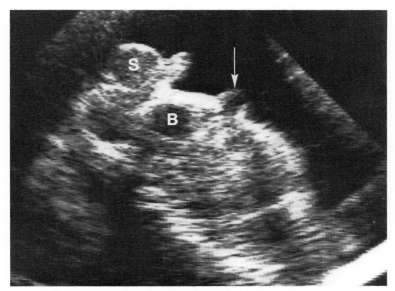

**Fig 8–4.**—Male, 34 weeks. Midline sagittal section through the trunk. The fetal scrotum *(S)* and penis can be appreciated, well separated from the insertion of the umbilical cord *(arrow).* *B* = Bladder.

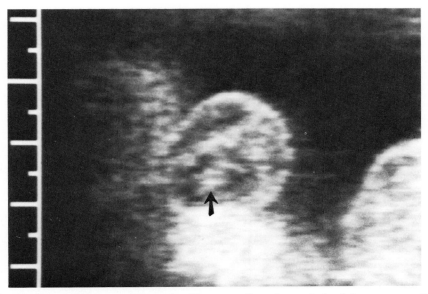

**Fig 8–5.**—Undescended testis, 35 weeks. Fetal scrotum delineates presence of only one, typically echogenic, testicle *(arrow).* The opposite side of the scrotum can be seen to be empty with no similar echogenic testicle identified. The testicle descent into the scrotum usually occurs during the seventh gestational month. By the eighth month, echogenic testicles are usually identified in both sides of the scrotum. While there may be some variation from side to side in timing of descent, failure to identify normal testicular tissue on both sides of the scrotum should be followed up after birth.

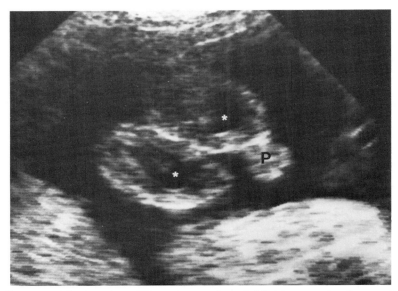

**Fig 8–6.**—Congenital hydroceles, 37 weeks. Transverse section through the scrotum and penis *(P)* reveals small bilateral hydroceles *(\*)* around the testicles. The isolated finding of hydroceles is a normal fetal variant. Small amounts of scrotal fluid may enter the scrotum at the time of testicular descent. With no decrease in the amount of fluid beyond that initially seen or the presence of associated peritoneal fluid, the potential for an inguinal hernia must be considered.

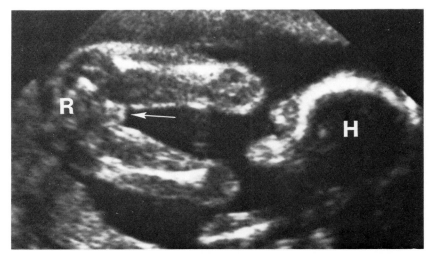

**Fig 8–7.**—Female, 22 weeks. Transverse section through the fetal pelvis and flexed thighs reveals female genitalia with the bilobed labia majora apparent *(arrow)*. H = head. R = rump.

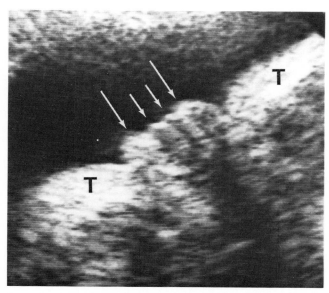

**Fig 8–8.**—Coronal section through the female genitalia at 34 weeks reveals the larger, lateral labia majora *(long arrows)* and the two smaller, medial labia minora *(short arrows). T* = thighs.

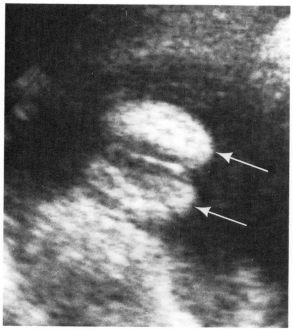

**Fig 8–9.**—Transverse section through the female genitalia at 37 weeks demonstrates the prominent labia majora *(arrows)* surrounding the less pronounced labia minora. The labia majora can become quite prominent, particularly in the third trimester. The male scrotum may be simulated; however, attention to the delineation of the smaller labium minora centrally and the lack of differentiation of the echogenic testicle within each side of the expected hemiscrotum should aid in differentiation.

REFERENCES

Birnholz J.C.: Determination of fetal sex. *N. Engl. J. Med.* 309:942–944, 1983.

Conrad A.R., Rao S.A.S.: Ultrasound diagnosis of fetal hydrocele. *Radiology* 127:232, 1978.

Dunne M.G., Cunat J.S.: Sonographic determination of fetal gender before 25 weeks gestation. *A.J.R.* 140:741–743, 1983.

Meizner I., Katz M., Zmora E., et al.: In utero diagnosis of congenital hydrocele. *J. C. U.* 11:449–450, 1983.

Scholly T.A., Sutphen J.H., Hitchcock D.A., et al.: Sonographic determination of fetal gender. *A.J.R.* 135:1161–1165, 1980.

Schotten A., Giese C.: The "female echo": prenatal determination of the female fetus by ultrasound. *Am. J. Obstet. Gynecol.* 138:463–464, 1980.

Shalev E., Weiner E., Zuckerman H.: Ultrasound determination of fetal sex. *Am. J. Obstet. Gynecol.* 141:582–583, 1981.

# CHAPTER 9

# Extremities

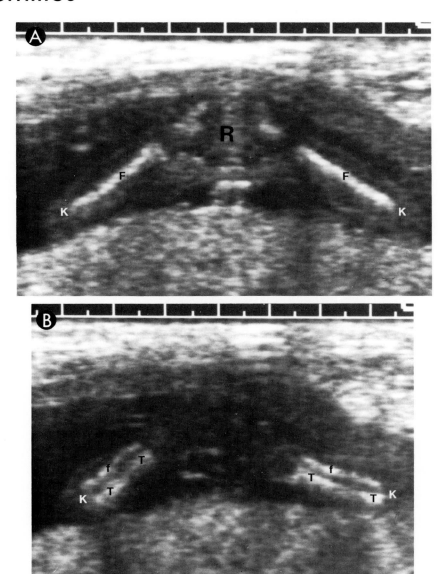

**Fig 9–1.**—Lower extremities, 17 weeks. Simultaneous imaging of the thighs **(A)** and legs **(B)** of a fetus in a prone position with the lower extremities abducted. The rump *(R)*, femurs *(F)*, tibias *(T)*, fibulas *(f)*, and region of the knee *(K)* are indicated. Such images that show several bones simultaneously are useful for rapid surveys of general fetal skeletal anatomy; however, if accurate measurements are required, individual bones should be imaged.

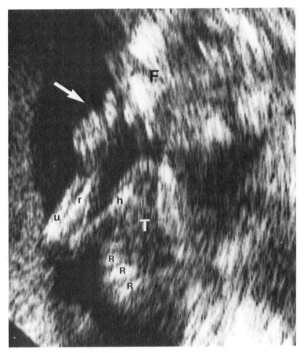

**Fig 9–2.**—Upper extremity, 17 weeks. Parasagittal image demonstrates a clenched fist, except for an extended index finger *(arrow)* anterior to the fetal face *(F)*. Parts of the forearm (*u* = ulna, *r* = radius) and arm (*h* = humerus) are seen anterior to the thorax. *R* = ribs. This fetus may well be a librarian someday.

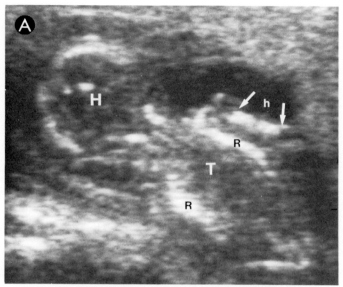

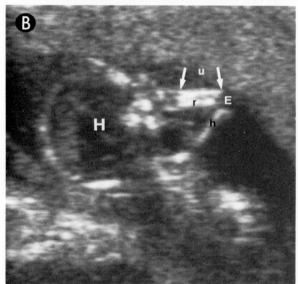

**Fig 9–3.**—Upper extremity long bones, 11 weeks. The fetal humerus *(h, arrows)* measures 10 mm and the ulna *(u, arrows)* measures 9 mm. The fetal radius *(r)* is slightly shorter than the ulna. The more proximal origination of the ulna within the elbow *(E),* and the nearly even point of distal termination of the radius and ulna are apparent even at this early stage of development. The fetal hand is near the face. *H* = head, *T* = thorax, with ribs *(R)* noted laterally.

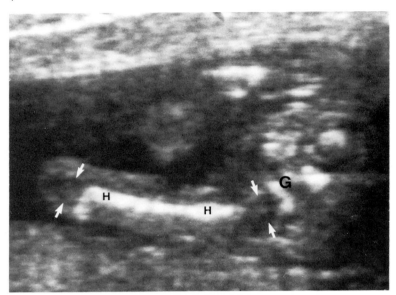

**Fig 9–4.**—Humerus, 15 weeks. The humerus *(H)* is identified by its position adjacent to the bones of the upper thorax and shoulder girdle *(G)*. Nonossified cartilage *(arrows)* within the humeral head and distal humerus is hypoechoic relative to adjacent soft tissue.

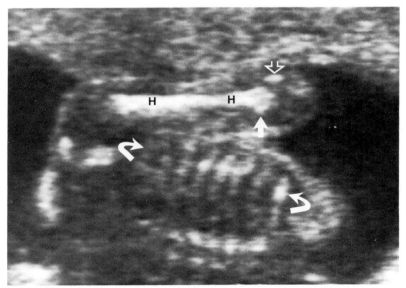

**Fig 9–5.**—Humerus, 19 weeks. Longitudinal image. The humerus *(H)* can be differentiated from the femur by identification of the adjacent shoulder girdle and ribs *(curved arrows)*. Note the mild flaring of the distal humerus at the level of the condyles *(solid arrow)*. A bright specular echo *(open arrow)* represents a lateral cutaneous margin, not a bone.

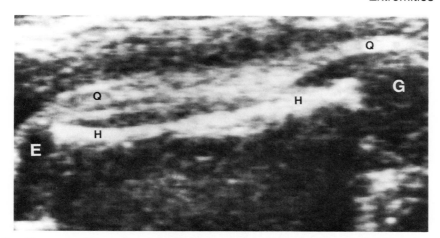

**Fig 9–6.**—Humerus, 33 weeks. Longitudinal image of the humerus *(H)* demonstrates a similarity to the appearance of the fetal femur, including a mild normal curvature. Hypoechoic musculature of the shoulder girdle *(G)* and elbow *(E)* are present deep to echogenic skin/subcutaneous tissue *(Q)*.

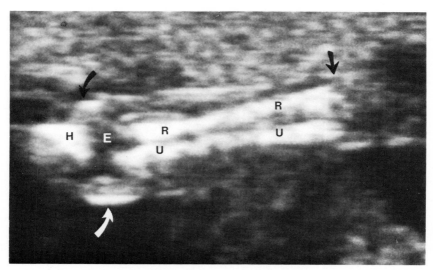

**Fig 9–7.**—Forearm, elbow, 20 weeks. The forearm can be localized by scanning to the distal humerus *(H)* and rotating the transducer through the elbow *(E)* to image the radius *(R)* and ulna *(U)*. The ulna is identified by its more proximal extent, while both radius and ulna terminate at approximately the same level within the wrist *(straight arrow)*. Imaging of the radius, in particular its distal extent, may be important in the various syndromes with radial dysplasia. *Curved arrows* indicate bright specular echoes from skin-fluid interfaces.

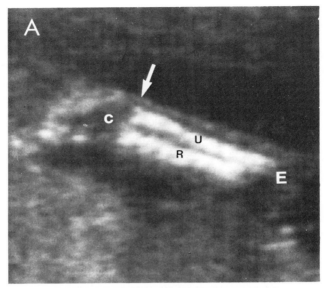

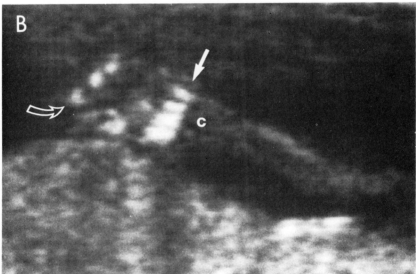

**Fig 9–8.**—Forearm, metacarpals, 15 weeks. **A,** distal radius *(R)* and ulna *(U)* terminate at approximately the same point within the wrist *(C),* whereas the proximal ulna extends further into the elbow *(E)* than the radius. The wrist is flexed on the forearm, making simultaneous coronal imaging of the hand and forearm impossible. **B,** an-gling of the transducer is necessary to image the metacarpals *(straight arrow),* the longest of which measures 4 mm. No ossified carpal bones are seen in utero *(C),* while portions of several ossified digits are present within a clenched fist *(curved arrow).*

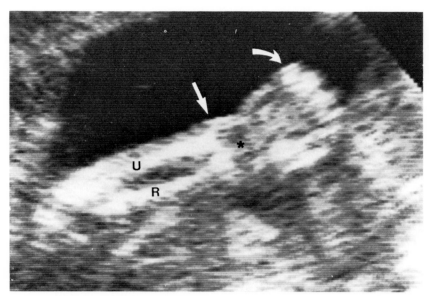

**Fig 9–9.**—Wrist. Longitudinal section demonstrates the radius *(R)* and ulna *(U)* terminating at the same approximate level *(straight arrow)*. The bones of the fetal wrist *(\*)* are generally not ossified in utero. The metacarpals are out of the plane of section; however, ossification centers within several phalanges can be appreciated *(curved arrow)*.

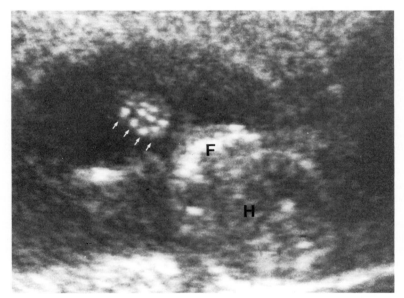

**Fig 9–10.**—Fingers, 14 weeks. Individual phalanges of several fingers *(arrows)* are imaged anterior to the face *(F)*. Each ossification center is only about 1.5 mm in size. *H* = head.

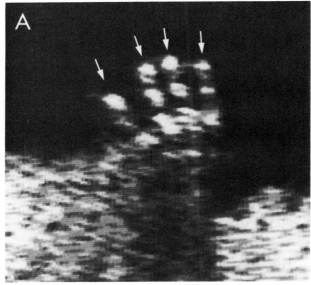

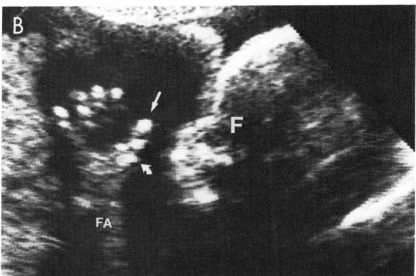

**Fig 9–11.**—Finger and thumb, 17.5 weeks. **A,** three individual phalanges of the extended fingers are identified *(arrows)*. **B,** transducer has been rotated to show the shorter thumb *(straight arrow)* and parts of all four fingers extended in front of the face *(F)*. The thumb has only two phalangeal ossification centers, adjacent to a portion of the first metacarpal *(curved arrow)*. Individual ossification centers measure 2.5–3 mm at this age. *FA* = forearm. Imaging the extended digits is difficult as the fetus frequently holds the hand in a clenched fist. The velocity with which any fetal part moves is also increased the further distally one moves, making the hands (and feet) two of the most difficult areas to "map out."

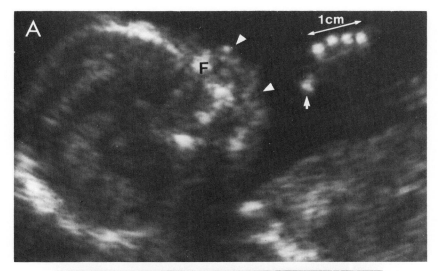

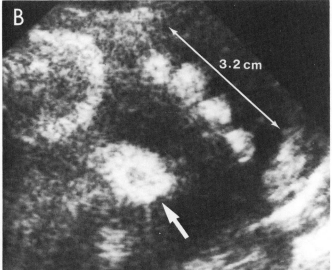

**Fig 9–12.**—Fingers, cross-section, 16 and 33 weeks. Cross-sections through a partially clenched fist at **(A)** 16 weeks and **(B)** 33 weeks demonstrate the difference in the bulk of the soft tissues and bones of the four fingers *(indicated measurements)* and the thumb *(arrows)*. The face *(F)* is seen in profile, with the mouth and nose indicated by *arrowheads*.

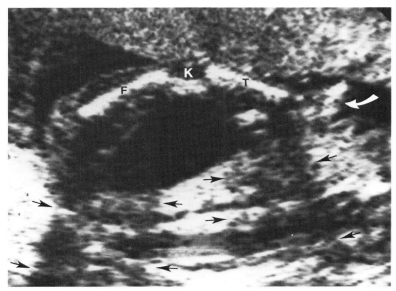

**Fig 9–13.**—Lower extremity, 18 weeks. A longitudinal image demonstrates the femur *(F)* within the thigh, separated from the tibia *(T)* by the hypoechoic knee *(K)*. Shadowing distal to the long bones is marked with *black arrows. White arrow* indicates the foot.

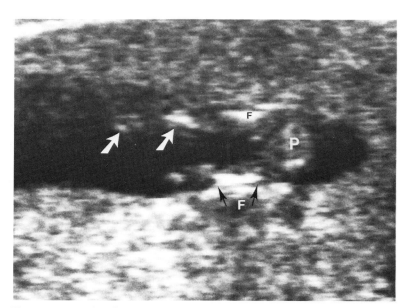

**Fig 9–14.**—Femur, 12 weeks. Section through the pelvis *(P)* and lower extremities demonstrates both femurs *(F). Black arrows* indicate only side satisfactory for measurement. A portion of the right leg and foot can be seen *(white arrows).* With optimal patient size, fetal position, and equipment, several major long bones may be imaged by 10–12 weeks gestational age.

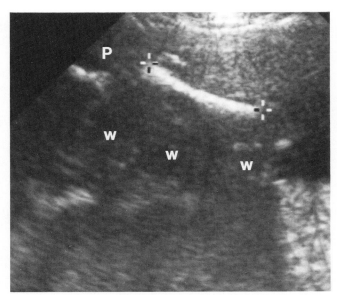

**Fig 9–15.**—Femur, 19 weeks. Electronic calipers *(+)* delineate the ends of the femur for measurement, indicating a length of 32 mm. A relatively uniform distal shadow *(W)* is desirable for optimal bone mensuration. *P* = proximal.

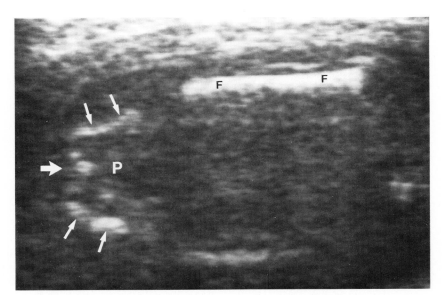

**Fig 9–16.**—Femur, 21 weeks. The femur is best localized by scanning transversely through the pelvis until the thighs are reached and the femur seen, followed by the appropriate rotation to obtain a longitudinal section of the femur. In this instance, the thigh is flexed on the pelvis *(P)* such that a longitudinal section of femur *(F)* is apparent simultaneously with a transverse image through the sacral spine *(wide arrow)* and iliac crests *(thin arrows)*.

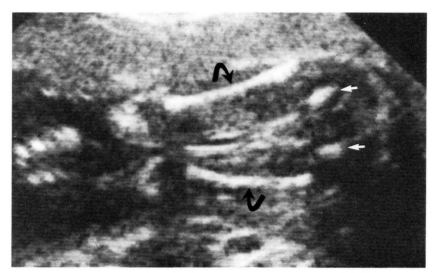

**Fig 9–17.**—Femurs. The ossification centers of the ischii *(white arrows)* will be the most frequently identified bony pelvic landmark when imaging the femurs *(curved arrows)*. Measured lengths of these femurs are several millimeters apart, and only the near one should be used for a femur length determination. Shadowing by the near femur or foreshortening due to difficulty in simultaneously imaging the maximal length of both bones makes it necessary to image only one for measurement.

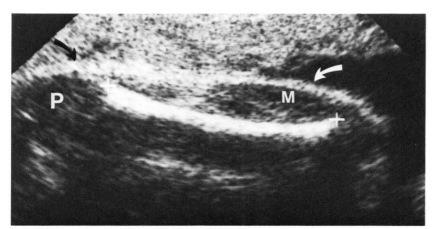

**Fig 9–18.**—Physiologic femur bowing, 26 weeks. Longitudinal image demonstrates slight normal physiologic bowing of the femur. Normal skin thickness is identified at this gestational age as a single echogenic line of approximately 1.5– 2 mm in thickness *(arrows)*, external to the hypoechoic musculature *(M)* surrounding the femur. Electronic calipers *(+)* indicate a femur length of 49 mm. *P* = proximal.

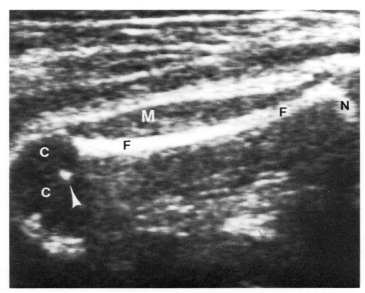

**Fig 9–19.**—Distal femoral epiphysis, 33 weeks. Longitudinal scan of the femur *(F)* delineates the small, echogenic, distal femoral epiphyseal ossification center (arrowhead). The ossification center lies within a larger mass of nonossified cartilage *(C)* which is more hypoechoic than muscle *(M)*. The femoral neck *(N)* can be appreciated proximally. The presence of the distal femoral ossification center indicates a gestational age of 33 or more weeks.

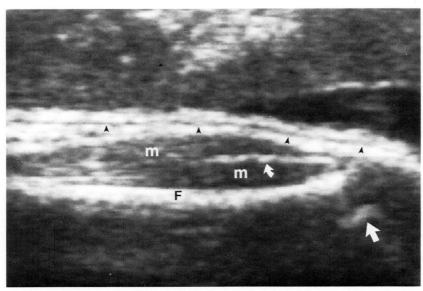

**Fig 9–20.**—Skin/subcutaneous thigh tissues, 37 weeks. Longitudinal section demonstrates the distal femoral epiphysis *(straight arrow)*, indicating at least a 33-week gestation. The previously uniformly echogenic skin/subcutaneous tissues (Fig 9–18) now show an approximately 1- 1.5-mm central sonolucent band *(arrowheads)*, representing increased subcutaneous fat stores as term is approached. The hypoechoic musculature of the thigh *(m)* is noted with an intervening echogenic fascial plane distally *(curved arrow).* F indicates fascia.

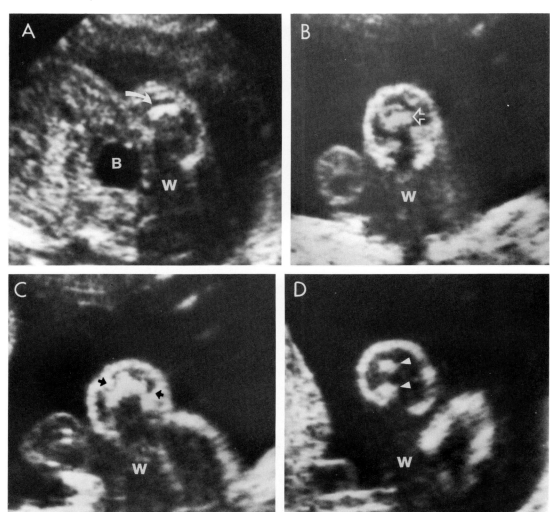

**Fig 9–21.**—Lower extremity, transverse sections, late second trimester. Sequential images through the thigh **(A–C)** and leg **(D)** demonstrate cross-sectional anatomy of the long bones. **A,** femoral neck *(curved arrow)* is seen in lengthwise section extending toward the pelvis *(B = bladder).* It is wider than the femoral shaft *(open arrow),* seen as a single central bone in the mid-thigh in **B. B,** femoral shaft *(open arrow).* **C,** distal femur has a V-shape *(short arrows)* representing the femoral condyles directed posteriorly. **D,** in contrast to the thigh, a cross-section through the leg reveals two long bones *(arrowheads)* with the mid-shaft of the tibia more centrally located than the fibula. At each level, the bones are surrounded by hypoechoic musculature which is in turn covered by the brightly echogenic skin and subcutaneous tissue which measures 2–3 mm. *W* = shadow.

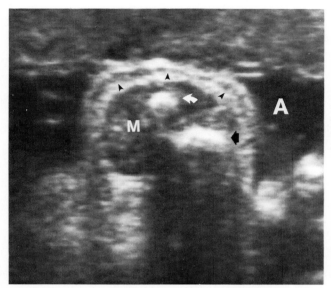

**Fig 9–22.**—Proximal leg, transverse, late third trimester. A transverse section demonstrates the wider appearance of the anteriorly positioned, tibial plateau/neck *(straight arrow)* and smaller size of the posterolateral fibular head *(curved arrow).* Note the prominence of the sonolucent subcutaneous fat *(arrowheads)* near term. *M* = musculature. *A* = anterior.

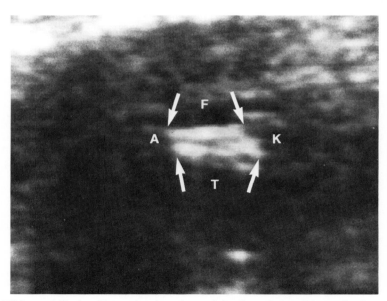

**Fig 9–23.**—Tibia and fibula, 10 weeks. Longitudinal scan of a 7-mm fibula *(F, arrows)* and 8-mm tibia *(T, arrows)* at 10 weeks. Note that even at this early stage of gestation, the more proximal origination of the tibia at the knee *(K)* and distal extent of the fibula at the ankle *(A)* can be appreciated.

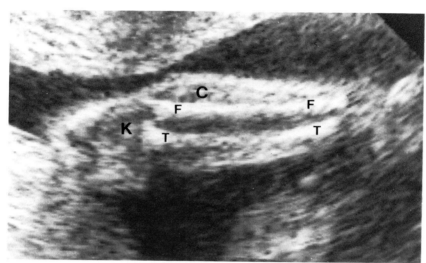

**Fig 9–24.**—Leg, 22 weeks. Longitudinal image demonstrates both the fibula *(F)* and tibia *(T).* The tibia is seen to extend further into the knee *(K),* while the fibula extends further at the ankle. For specific long bone measurements, selected images of individual bones are suggested (Fig 9–25). However, for orientation and delineating anatomic relationships between bones, such simultaneous imaging is useful. The soft tissues of the calf *(C)* are noted to be fuller than those of the ankle.

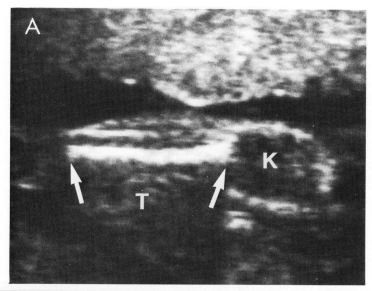

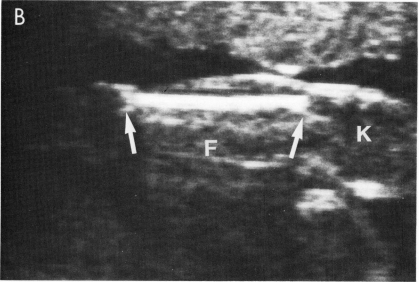

**Fig 9–25.**—Tibia and fibula, 21 weeks. Select **(A)** tibia and **(B)** fibula measurements at 21 weeks. The tibia *(T, arrows)* measures 34 mm and is more centrally located within the leg than the fibula *(F, arrows)*, which measures 33 mm. Note the echogenic, thick image of each bone with well-defined ends and good distal shadowing, as contrasted with simultaneously imaged bones in Figure 9–24. *K* = knee.

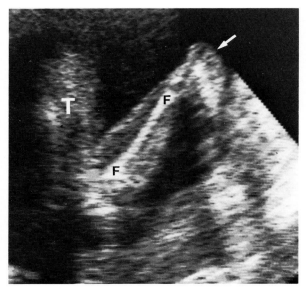

**Fig 9–26.**—Fibula, 16 weeks. A long section of fibula *(F)* is identified within the soft tissues of the leg. Relationships with the thigh *(T)* and the foot *(arrow)* flexed on the leg are noted.

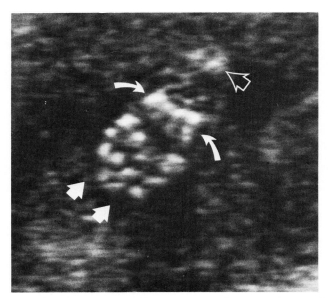

**Fig 9–27.**—Foot, 17 weeks. Axial image delineates multiple phalanges *(closed arrows)* and metatarsals *(curved arrows)*, as well as a portion of the calcaneus *(open arrow)*.

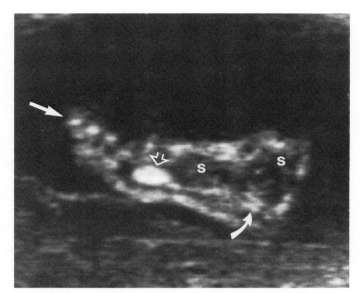

**Fig 9–28.**—Foot, 27 weeks. Sagittal section demonstrates the phalanges in a single ray *(straight arrow)*, a portion of one metatarsal *(open arrow)*, part of the calcaneus *(curved arrow)*, and soft tissues within the foot and ankle *(S)*.

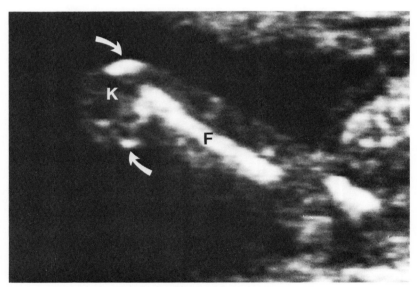

**Fig 9–29.**—Pitfall, bone identification. Longitudinal image of the femur *(F)*. Bright specular echoes *(arrows)* superficially at the knee *(K)* represent only amniotic fluid-skin surface interfaces and should not be mistaken for osseous structures.

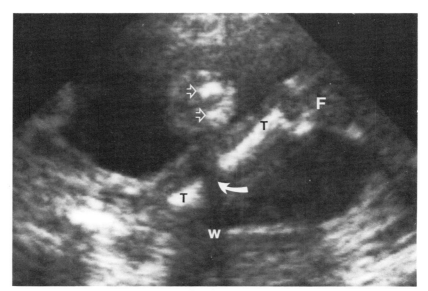

**Fig 9–30.**—Pitfall, bone length and continuity, 20 weeks. Apparent discontinuity in the tibia *(T)* *(curved arrow)* is caused by shadowing *(W)* from the long bones of the opposite leg *(open arrows)*. Care should be taken to image all bones free of shadowing from proximal structures so that foreshortening or apparent discontinuities are not created. F = foot.

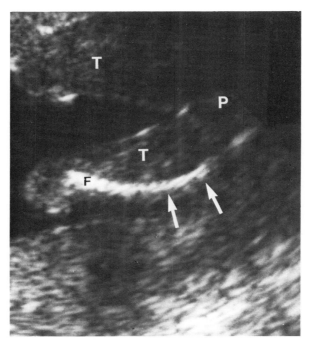

**Fig 9–31.**—Pitfall, excessive femur bowing, 18 weeks. Technically inadequate femur *(F)* with apparent pronounced bowing. The proximal shaft *(arrows)* is tapered in configuration, is less reflective, and causes less shadowing than the distal shaft, indicating only partial imaging of the proximal portion. Repeat imaging with the scanning plane altered to demonstrate a uniformly thick and echogenic femur revealed mild physiologic bowing only. *P* = pelvis. *T* = soft tissue of thighs.

152

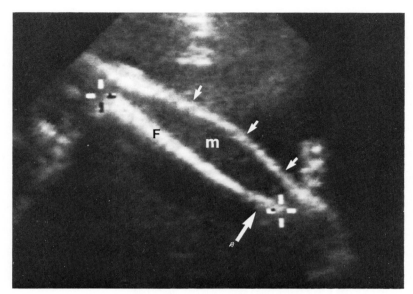

**Fig 9–32.**—Pitfall, femur mensuration, 27 weeks. The electronically measured (+) femur is suboptimal since the tapered configuration and reduced echo amplitude of the distal femur *(long arrow)* suggest a foreshortened measurement. *m* = muscle mass. *Short arrows* indicate normal subcutaneous tissue/skin thickness for age.

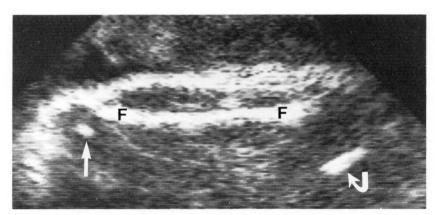

**Fig 9–33.**—Pitfall, differentiation of distal femoral epiphysis from the ischial ossification, 35 weeks. Longitudinal image through the femur *(F)* delineates the distal femoral epiphysis *(straight arrow)*. The close proximity of the epiphysis to the distal femur is contrasted with a greater separation between the ischial ossification center *(curved arrow)* and the proximal of the femur. If routine transverse imaging through the abdomen to the bony pelvis is performed prior to imaging the femur, no difficulty in differentiating proximal and distal femur should occur.

REFERENCES

Chinn D.H., Bolding D.B., Callen P.W., et al.: Ultrasonographic identification of fetal lower extremity epiphyseal ossification centers. *Radiology* 147:815–818, 1983.

Farrant P., Meire H.B.: Ultrasound measurement of fetal limb lengths. *Br. J. Radiol.* 54:660–664, 1981.

Filly R.A., Golbus M.S.: Ultrasonography of the normal and pathologic fetal skeleton, Symposium on Ultrasonography in Obstetrics and Gynecology. *Radiol. Clin. North Am.* 20:311–323, 1982.

Filly R.A., Golbus M.S., Carey J.C., et al.: Short-limbed dwarfism: ultrasonographic diagnosis by mensuration of fetal femoral length. *Radiology* 138:653–656, 1981.

Gentili P., Trasimeni A., Giorlandino C.: Fetal ossification centers as predictors of gestational age in normal and abnormal pregnancies. *J. Ultrasound Med.* 3:193–197, 1984.

Hadlock F.P., Deter R.L., Roecker E., et al.: Relation of fetal femur length to neonatal crown-heel length. *J. Ultrasound Med.* 3:1–3, 1984.

Hadlock F.P., Harrist R.B., Deter R.L., et al.: Fetal femur length as a predictor of menstrual age: sonographically measured. *A.J.R.* 138:875–878, 1982.

Hadlock F.P., Harrist R.B., Shah Y., et al.: The femur length/head circumference relation in obstetric sonography. *J. Ultrasound Med.* 3:439–442, 1984.

Hobbins J.C., Bracken M.B., Mahoney M.J.: Diagnosis of fetal skeletal dysplasias with ultrasound. *Am. J. Obstet. Gynecol.* 142:306–312, 1982.

Hohler C.W., Quetel T.A.: Comparison of ultrasound femur length and biparietal diameter in late pregnancy. *Am. J. Obstet. Gynecol.* 141:759–762, 1981.

Hohler C.W., Quetel T.A.: Fetal femur length: equations for computer calculation of gestational age from ultrasound measurements. *Am. J. Obstet. Gynecol.* 143:479–481, 1982.

Jeanty P., Dramaix-Wilmet M., van Kerkem J., et al.: Ultrasonic evaluation of fetal limb growth. *Radiology* 143:751–754, 1982.

Jeanty P., Kirkpatrick C., Dramaix-Wilmet M., et al.: Ultrasonic evaluation of fetal limb growth. *Radiology* 140:165–168, 1981.

Jeanty P., Rodesch F., Delbeke D., et al.: Estimation of gestational age from measurements of fetal long bones. *J. Ultrasound Med.* 3:75–79, 1984.

Mahony B.S., Filly R.A.: High-resolution sonographic assessment of the fetal extremities. *J. Ultrasound Med.* 3:489–498, 1984.

McLeary R.D., Kuhns L.R.: Sonographic evaluation of the distal femoral epiphyseal ossification center. *J. Ultrasound Med.* 2:437–438, 1983.

O'Brien G.D., Queenan J.T.: Growth of the ultrasound fetal femur length during normal pregnancy. *Am. J. Obstet. Gynecol.* 141(pt. 1):833–837, 1981.

O'Brien G.D., Queenan J.T., Campbell S.: Assessment of gestational age in the second trimester by real-time ultrasound measurement of the femur length. *Am. J. Obstet. Gynecol.* 139:540–545, 1981.

Quinlan R.W., Brumfield C., Martin M., et al.: Ultrasonic measurement of femur length as a predictor of fetal gestational age. *J. Reprod. Med.* 27:392–394, 1982.

Wong W.S., Filly R.A.: Polyhydramnios associated with fetal limb abnormalities. *A.J.R.* 140:1001–1003, 1983.

Yeh M., Bracero L., Reilly K.B., et al.: Ultrasonic measurement of the femur length as an index of fetal gestational age. *Am. J. Obstet. Gynecol.* 144:519–522, 1982.

# Index

**155**